MW01615251

POWER COUPLE

HABITS

DR. SCOTT AND AMY NOORDA

This book is dedicated to the many vibrant examples of inspired and powerful relationships that we have been privileged to learn from.

And to our children, that they may learn how to live their best lives from the very beginning.

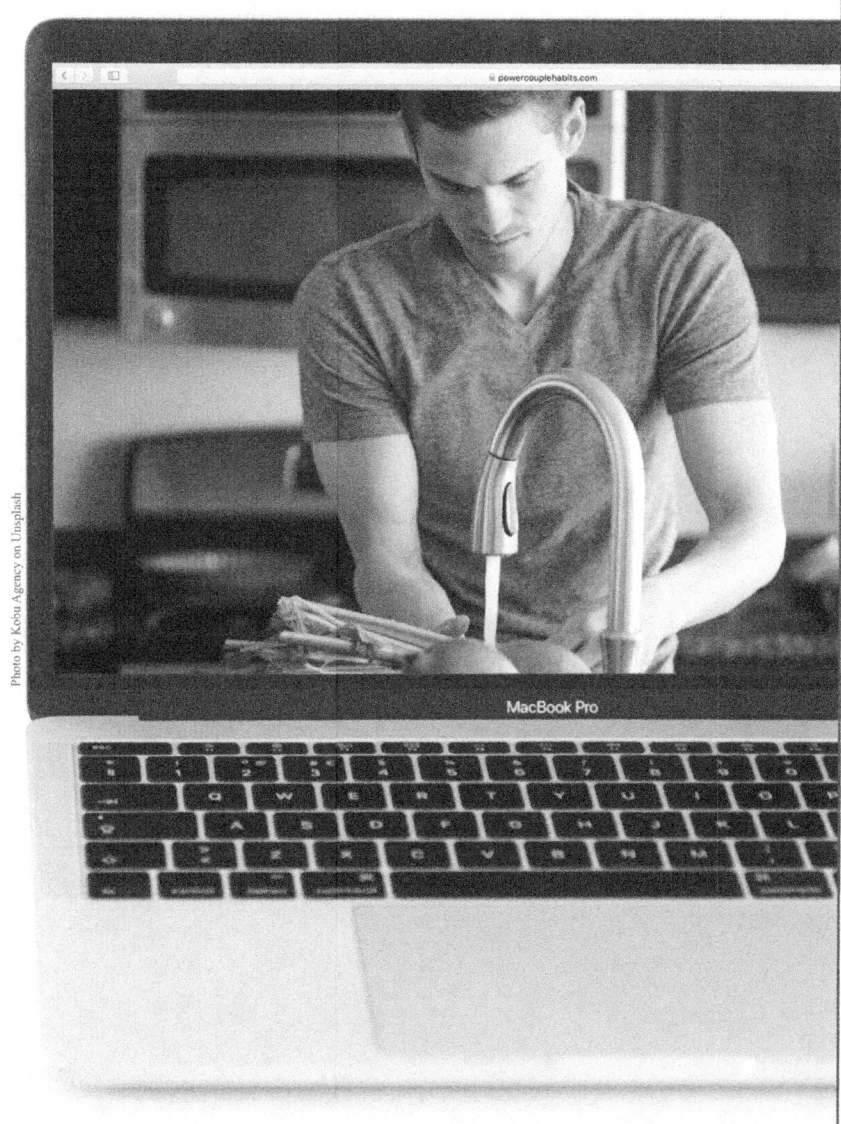

free downloads at
powercouplehabits.com/gift

CONTENTS

PART 3: STRESS

PART 4: PURPOSE + COMMITMENT

PART 5: RELATIONSHIP

FINAL THOUGHTS

POWER COUPLE HABITS

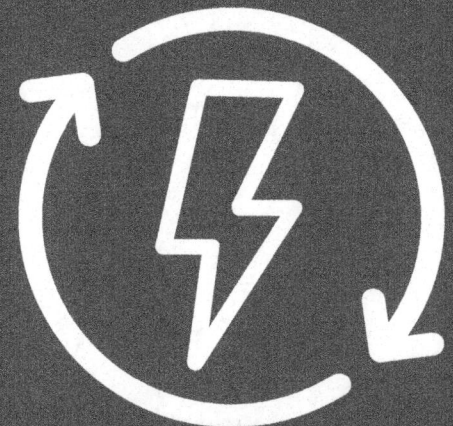

POWER UP

The more you
align the things
you DO with
the things
you DESIRE,
the more power
you invite into
your life.

JUST LIKE EVERY OTHER DAY, Dad gave my bike one last push before we made it to the last downhill leg of our daily ride to school and then started jogging to keep up as I raced down. I smiled back at him, the most carefree boy in the world.

This memory is one of my "Peter Pan" happy thoughts.

It wasn't until years later that I realized that Dad was much more tired than I was when he was giving me a boost on my bike. He worked swing shift and didn't get to bed until after 2 AM, but was still up first thing in the morning, getting us off to school. He never once complained about pushing my bike along or chasing me down the hill—I'm not sure which one was more exhausting!

My dad worked hard. In addition to his engineering job at the Air Force Base, he spent every other weekend working for the Army National Guard. And on top of all that, he maintained the cherry orchard next to our house—beehives and all.

My dad was incredibly selfless. In fact, he rarely even talked about himself. As a young adult I realized that I didn't know very much about my Dad. I figured I would have time later in life to get to know him better.

Unfortunately, that never really happened.

Not too many years later, my dad was on another downhill path. Within a few years of his retirement, Alzheimer's began to steal his identity, his personality, and his memories.

By the time I had the tools to help him, it was too late.

I would give anything to back his life up 20 years. With that time I could decrease the odds of his current outcome dramatically.

It's amazing what an understanding of genetics, nutrition, lifestyle, environmental toxins, and relationships can do in the fight against Alzheimer's. Research showing prevention (and even reversal in some cases) through advanced lifestyle interventions is extremely promising.

As I ran alongside my kids on their way to school the other day I was reminded of those special moments with my dad.

My dad isn't even able to walk down the sidewalk with his grand kids anymore, but I am living each day with the goal to optimize my health so that I can be present and active for my children and future grandchildren.

This is what motivates Amy and me to continue to push ourselves each day to study, live, and teach the ways Alzheimer's disease and other chronic diseases can be prevented and more effectively treated.

Most chronic diseases are caused by a combination of genetic risk factors and environmental triggers. But it's not as much about your genes as you think. Your lifestyle and environment account for up to 95% of your risk for chronic illness.[1]

**SO, YOU WANT (NEED!) TO BE HEALTHIER,
BUT WHERE DO YOU START?**

You want more energy, to think more clearly, and to look and feel better.

And you are highly motivated to avoid the chronic illnesses you see in your friends, family, and in your own future.

But it is overwhelming to figure out how to get there.

In a world of information overload, it's hard to find trustworthy advice on a topic surrounded by misinformation. Once you find accurate information, there is so much to learn and do differently that you may get overwhelmed and put it off. How do you add life-altering to-dos to a list that is already running off the page?

You are who we write for.

We research extensively—reading medical journals and published literature, as well as learning from the experience of other physicians. We've sifted through the information and are ready to share the results in a method that will empower you to act.

We've been studying how to live healthier for years. Even after seven years of medical school and training, I still felt like I didn't have the tools to address the underlying lifestyle and environmental causes of chronic conditions. This led me to do extensive post-graduate training on the physiology and biology of disease and the pathway to health.

Amy and I are on our own health journey and we have the privilege of observing many other health journeys—both in clinical practice and with friends and family.

As a Family Medicine physician with experience working in the hospital and in private practice, I consistently see that the individuals who are the most successful in making sustainable lifestyle changes are those who change with their spouse. A couple will often have a similar "WHY"—a motivating factor that unites them as they plan, work, and celebrate together on their unique health journey.

We have observed attributes and habits of strong, healthy, successful couples and identified common elements that exist in varying degrees in each Power Couple we know. These are 100% attainable habits and traits.

Above all, we want to empower you to work together to live your best life and we're going to help you do it one step at a time.

In this book, we share some of the steps that I walk my patients through to maintain—or regain—their trajectory. A high-achieving mindset is all about maximizing growth. Incorporating these habits ensures that you keep gaining. Even better, you're doing it together.

This isn't just another self-help book, it's a couple-upgrade book.

We'll share real-world examples and experience gained from interaction with thousands of patients. We'll show how utilizing the power of habits and working together to make lifestyle changes can take you to the next level in your health, your work, and your relationship.

Perfection Pending

It's important for you to realize that we are not perfect in these things. We often struggle with meal planning. One of us (OK, Amy) is still working on willfully going outside during the winter—no matter how badly vitamin D is needed! And we disregarded all the science and were sitting at our computers into the late hours of the night when we were finishing up the last section of this book—conveniently not the sleep section!

We're not perfect and you won't be either. What's most important is that you are inspired to do a little better today than you did yesterday. If you can get to where you are reaching your eating, sleeping, and de-stressing goals 51% of the time, then you have tipped the scales in your favor!

Each of these challenges should be something that you work on together. The power of two is strong. Be bold in committing.

Here's to being better together and a better tomorrow.

2 SECRETS TO
SUSTAINABLE

CHANGE

1. CHANGE WITH SOMEONE YOU LOVE.

....

2. MAKE HARD CHANGES EASIER BY CREATING HABITS.

1. CHANGE WITH SOMEONE YOU LOVE.

Working together is more fun than working alone.

Accountability, partnership, encouragement, inspiration…these are all powerful things that come from working with somebody else.

When you want to implement powerful change in your life, who better to do that with than the partner you have chosen to go through life with?

Not every power couple does all the things that we outline in this book. Some master one or two sections and are happy with the success it brings to their lives. Some people do a little bit of all of them and love the changes that they see.

The key is to recognize where you are misaligned—to define what is holding you back from who you want to be and what you want to achieve—and then attack those things together, one-by-one, always with a patient (but determined) plan for progression.

2. MAKE HARD CHANGES EASIER BY CREATING HABITS.

Performance science teaches us that it takes more than just motivation to change how we think and what we do. Motivation is as fluid as the tide—we start out strong, but it's often gone by early afternoon.

If we want to effect real (i.e. consistent) change in our lives, we need to get scientific. We can hack our brains to make our desired actions unconscious—things we do without having to think about them.

Neuroscience entrepreneur and biohacker, James Garrett, teaches that habits are responsible for 40-50% of our daily behavior. He explains that our brains are energy-efficient habit-making machines that detect patterns in our behavior and then outsource those actions to the subconscious.

While decisions require a constant refueling of attention and energy, habits move you into energy-efficient autopilot mode.

However, a habit is not a quick fix. As James Garrett puts it, "Habits are slow and steady, not flashy. Habits happen over time."[2]

It's important to recognize that you don't just want quick fix solutions to your problems. What you really want is life-long sustainable improvement.

Optimal health and true healing require effort.

Change that will last over time requires an investment of time.

In fact, we believe that our purpose for living is to invest time—our lifetime—in learning how to change for the better.

Stephen R. Covey revolutionized the self-help world thirty years ago with his focus on principle-centered habits in *The 7 Habits of Highly Effective People*. In this timeless work, he defines the relationship between habits and power, saying:

> Power is the faculty or capacity to act, the strength
> and potency to accomplish something. It is the vital
> energy to make choices and decisions. It also includes
> the capacity to overcome deeply embedded habits and
> to cultivate higher, more effective ones.[3]

Our purpose for living
is to invest time—our
lifetime—in learning
how to change for
the better.

When we are willing to act—to change and grow—we draw power into all facets of our lives: physical, mental, spiritual, and social. As we strive to realign our daily thoughts and actions to our principles, we become truly powerful.

In the chapters that follow, you will find suggestions for habits that will give you greater health and power.

As you work together to gain new habits and achieve new goals, you will find overall fulfillment, greater control of your outcomes, and ultimately, more zest for all the great things life has to offer.

WHAT IS A POWER COUPLE?

Some might say that it's the latest celebrity hook-up. Others might point to political powerhouses, flourishing philanthropists, or dynamic business duos.

We're going for a little bit more depth in our definition:

SYNERGISTIC
They achieve so much more working together than they can individually. 1 + 1 = so much more than 2!

SUCCESSFUL
They are successful in the areas of life that matter most. (Spoiler Alert: it's not wealth, status, or social media followers).

STRONG
Their relationship gives them confidence. They are resilient, brave, and they do hard things together!

BALANCED
They protect priorities and develop talents in multiple areas. They emphasize healthy and clean living.

Simply put, being a Power Couple means being a combined force for good. Together, they bring life and light wherever they go.

So how do they do it? More importantly, how do YOU do it?

5 WAYS TO HELP YOUR SPOUSE GET ON BOARD WITH CHANGE

1. Focus on the Future

Talk together about your long-term vision and discuss how you can set yourselves up to be healthy enough to live the life you want in 10, 20, and 30+ years.

Keep everything positive and future-oriented instead of focusing on the process. Always bring it back to that picture of your ideal life together.

Instead of saying, "You need to stop drinking soda every day!" try: "After our date Friday let's stop at Whole Foods and pick up a couple new drinks to try that might be better for us than soda."

2. Create the Win

Everybody likes a little motivation.

A successful entrepreneurial couple shared with us the idea of a "90-Day Push". When they set a goal or plan a big project, they use a getaway trip as the reward. They dedicate themselves to working really hard for 90 days and have to meet their deadline because the trip is already planned!

You can set up your own 30, 60, or 90-day push. You and your spouse can pick a reward together or let your spouse pick the reward.

Choose a section to work on and create some great habits, looking ahead to your big win to keep you going.

3. Start with You

The best way to inspire change in others is to model that change in yourself. Showing is always better than telling!

If you start making changes and your spouse sees you having fun AND getting results, he/she will be much more excited to jump in.

4. Small Invitations

Your spouse might be nervous to change because he/she is afraid of failing or the commitment involved.

If your husband has always felt insecure in the kitchen, ask for help with a small job and then give him space to do it his way and ample gratitude and praise.

If your wife doesn't love spending time outdoors, find a short walk or hike with a beautiful view that makes it feel more worth it. Make it as special and as fun as you can—plan a picnic or some downtime in a secluded spot to just sit and talk or soak up some sun.

5. Gift It

Sometimes the hesitation is in not having the right tools.

Maybe some new running shoes would help motivate your spouse to join you on your evening jog.

A healthy cookbook with fabulous pictures might sway your significant other into discovering that healthy food is more than just steamed veggies.

Encouraging your spouse to experiment with a new super-powered blender might spark creativity in your morning smoothies.

When one area of your life is out of alignment, every area of your life suffers. You can't compartmentalize a working system. Although it's easy to push certain areas—like your health and relationships—to the side, you unwittingly infect your whole life. Eventually and always, the essentials you procrastinate or avoid will catch up to your detriment.

No matter where you are right now, you can have any future you want. But one thing is for certain, what you plant you must harvest. So, please plant with intention. Mental creation always precedes physical creation. The blueprint you design in your head becomes the life you build.[4]

BENJAMIN HARDY, ORGANIZATIONAL PSYCHOLOGIST AND BEST-SELLING AUTHOR

HOW TO USE THIS BOOK

In each of the following five sections you'll find five habits in each section that will help you uplevel your lifestyle to invite greater physical, mental, and spiritual health.

You can work your way through all of them or just choose the ones that will make the most difference for you.

Most people do best when they focus on one habit at a time.

If you're motivated to see bigger results faster, you can tackle a whole section (five habits) together.

Many of the habits work synergistically and can easily be combined, even between sections. For example: create a habit that combines exercise and nature, or nature and communication, or gratitude and journaling.

We've created a free action guide to help you complete the challenges that you can download from our website:

Resources available at
powercouplehabits.com

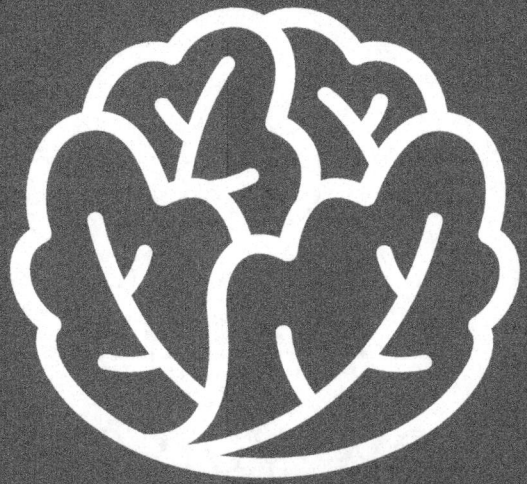

NUTRITION

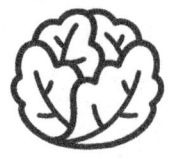

Changing
how you eat
will change
how well you
feel, think, look,
and perform.

EAT REAL FOOD

THE SINGLE LARGEST TRIGGER FOR ILLNESS is inferior nutrition. And it makes sense, right? We all know deep down that the things we put into our bodies either help them or hurt them.

Scott's alma mater, Brigham Young University, collaborated on a peer-reviewed study of 20,000 U.S. workers showing that those who ate healthy and exercised had 27% fewer sick days. According to the findings, "workers who ate healthy the entire day were 25% more likely to have higher job performance."[1]

Would you prefer to use your sick days for something other than being sick? Are you looking for ways to boost your productivity?

You need to fuel your body just like you fuel your car.

If you want high performance, you aren't buying watered-down gas from the corner pump because it's cheaper and more convenient— you're willing to go the extra mile (literally) to get high-octane fuel.

So, what does your body consider high-octane fuel? What should you be eating to minimize sick days and maximize performance?

Real food, eaten during real meals.

The answer is so simple that you almost feel silly saying it out loud, but it's become a real challenge in a world of microwave dinners, drive-thrus on every corner, dual-income families, and the dying art of truly enjoying food.

Our culture is fundamentally based on efficiency, leaving no room in most family schedules for a thoughtfully-prepared meal leisurely enjoyed around the dining table.

What have we lost in our quest for convenience and how badly do we want it back? What could possibly propel us into changing our food culture?

Motivating Change

We primarily see three motivating factors that drive lifestyle changes:

1. CHRONIC DISEASE

Autoimmune disease, diabetes, asthma, cancer, Alzheimer's... the number of people affected by chronic issues is staggering, but even more astounding is the rate at which the numbers are growing each year.

Research shows that the majority of chronic disease is caused by lifestyle choices.[2,3,4,5,6] A study looking at the effect diet has on the GI tract states,

Evidence suggests that the composition of the intestinal microbiota can influence susceptibility to chronic disease of the intestinal tract including ulcerative colitis, Crohn's disease, celiac disease and irritable bowel syndrome, as well as more systemic diseases such as obesity, type 1 diabetes and type 2 diabetes. Interestingly, a considerable shift in diet has coincided with increased incidence of many of these inflammatory diseases.[7]

You can live with a diagnosis for the rest of your life and take medications to try and mask symptoms (some with side effects worse than the illness itself!) or you can address the root cause of the problem and, in many cases, reverse the disease. For the people who come to us, changing the way they eat is a small price to pay for regaining their life.

2. LOSS OF PRODUCTIVITY AND MOMENTUM.

It's a story we hear over and over from entrepreneurs, business leaders, and high-level professionals. Work and life were great, but somehow fatigue and brain fog began creeping in, threatening to mess with their upward trajectory. Productivity is dropping at a nerve-wracking rate and work/life balance is becoming nonexistent.

We hear things like, "I'm in a funk, I just can't think as fast as I used to." or, "I'm tired all the time and by the end of the day I don't have any energy left to play with my kids."

A threat to your professional aspirations or your family life is enough to make lifestyle changes seem a lot more doable, and really… necessary.

3. REDISCOVERING PASSION

For many people, the drive to learn how to eat healthy comes when they have children and realize they want the best for them now and in the future. For some, watching a loved one experience health problems can be a catalyst for avoiding them in their own life. For others, an interest in nutrition accompanies a passion for learning about other health-related issues. And then there are the people whose motivation stems from a love of food and cooking.

Which of these reasons do you relate most to? We humans usually need a big reason to make a big change.

The first two motivations—chronic disease and loss of productivity and momentum—have urgency behind them that necessitates change. The third motivator—discovering or rediscovering a passion for health and food—is usually a slower, more scenic journey, and that has been our story.

OUR FOOD JOURNEY

Our initial motivation to cook was that we loved food and wanted to learn how to make it together. We weren't willing to learn as much from our parents during those teenage years as they wanted to teach us, and it wasn't until after we were married that we realized that if we still wanted to be able to enjoy all of those amazing baked goods that my mom used to make, we had better learn how to bake them on our own.

As newlyweds, we didn't feel like we knew how to cook much beyond the basics (i.e. pasta and quesadillas), but we loved eating good food and the budget just didn't allow for eating good food that other people cooked. So, we started learning together.

As we learned together, we also made it a point to try and learn from others and that was when the journey really took off.

BYU & BYU-Hawaii

In the early years of our marriage we were lucky enough to be surrounded by couples who came from all over the world to attend Brigham Young University, and later BYU-Hawaii for a few months. We learned how to cook Chinese food from the Qian and Ho families. We learned all about dim sum and how to make our own kimchi from Sun and Su.

The Galasos taught us how to make authentic empanadas and some other friends taught us about the beauty that is borscht. Andrew and Christina fueled our need for food-based adventures and later gave us the ultimate food tour of the Florida Keys.

Chicago

When we lived in Chicago, we learned all about using whole grains from our amazing friend, Angelika. Her traditional Austrian upbringing gave her an entirely different perspective on food and she taught us how to use different whole grains for different types of baking. We bought a countertop wheat grinder just like hers and it changed our lives. An added bonus: she showed us that a simple squeeze of lemon and drizzle of olive oil to dress a salad is tastier than a $4 bottle of salad dressing off the shelf.

Our next-door neighbors, Shannon and Writer, encouraged Scott's med-school coping mechanism: a new-found love for baking bread. Shannon taught me to appreciate Mexican food for breakfast (huevos rancheros for life!). John and Robin had marvelous potluck dinner parties in their beautiful backyard and encouraged a love of herbs, eating seasonally, and sustainable food sourcing.

Leanna taught us to cook beans and freeze them in 1 cup scoops to later throw into brownies, breads, or soups. Becca and Adam introduced us to the world of raw food sauces (almonds/chickpeas/tofu/lemon juice/spices/oh my!) when they showed us how to make the famous Eugene, Oregon favorite: Yumm Bowls. Our good friend, Nan, was great at having healthy snacks available for kids at all times and inspired us to do the same.

Nima took us downtown to experience Little India and instilled a passion for Indian food when she cooked with us in her house and ours. Another friend came to our home and taught us how to make Puerto Rican food and challenged us to eat whole garlic cloves raw (not for the faint of heart).

Jason and Becca took us to their favorite Pupuseria downtown and while the wives were busy chatting, the husbands talked the sweet grandmas working in the kitchen into a private pupusa lesson.

Houston

When we lived in Texas, Cristin taught us how easy (and delicious) it is to make your own almond milk and that you can make amazing treats using dates instead of sugar. She also showed us how to soak and dehydrate grains and nuts for greater nutrition—and better snacking! Her soaked and dehydrated buckwheat "croutons" are the best for enhancing a salad. Her husband, Jason, would whip up fresh garden salsas in an instant that our kids would devour even faster.

Tonya taught us how to make real food fit in a busy family schedule through planning, early preparation, and utilizing great tools, such as a crockpot. Another friend would prepare dinner right after breakfast so that her cooking and kitchen clean up would be finished by 9 AM.

Ben and Stacie were passionate about learning to cook international fare and were just as spontaneous as we were, leading to many amazing last-minute dinner parties. Kim's cheese-tasting nights helped expand our palettes and brought a new tradition to our holidays.

Raleigh

Our time in Raleigh further cemented our love of seafood and became the home base for a plethora of road trips to foodie hubs like Asheville, NOLA, and DC. Heidi and Monte encouraged a love of Southern BBQ. Katie taught us how to make one of our favorite dressings, a pear vinaigrette, and how important it is to empower our children in the kitchen. Rachel reminded us how much we love cold-pressed juice and inspired us to be more creative in our juicing.

Scott's bread baking talents transitioned to sourdough and adding more ancient grains (like einkorn wheat, teff, and kamut) to the repertoire, as well as using sprouted grains & flours in baking. We even sourced our own sprouted flour directly from a mill in Chapel Hill.

St. George

Another cross-country move brought new friends and new food. Laura encouraged an instant pot obsession and extended an unofficial Melissa Clark fan club invitation. (Real food recipes with fabulous photos...it was love at first sight.)[8] Monica and Devin taught us how to make authentic Japanese food. Anja modeled how to smoothly plan and cook for a crowd.

All of these places and friends (and so many more) were instrumental in developing our family's food culture and our passion for real food. Food became a foundation for friendships, a way to relax and destress, a reason to vacation (wait… who needs a reason?) and an enduring joy in our lives.

As we both studied and learned more about health (Scott via the traditional route of school, Amy via personal research), we recognized the clear correlation between quality of food and quality of life and became passionate about learning more.

We became champions of real milk (unpasteurized, non-homogenized) when one of our children experienced terrible eczema that didn't respond to conventional methods, but cleared instantly upon introducing raw goat's milk.

We studied everything that we could get our hands on to accompany our personal anecdotal experience and this led Scott to develop a graduate research project reviewing official recommendations on dairy consumption and actual in-practice dairy recommendations for children.

The passion was fueled even more as we realized how many people around us were struggling with autoimmune issues that could find relief by adjusting their lifestyles.

It became a personal mission for us to learn as much as we could and share that knowledge with people who are seeking solutions. These are usually people who have been to countless physicians and are truly desperate for answers. They've been told their disease is in their head, or that they need to take three medications to manage their disease and two more medications to manage the side effects.

When we share what we know, time and again these people return with tears in their eyes to tell us how grateful they are to feel well again and have their lives back.

The examples of these strong and persistent individuals we have the honor of working with motivates us even more to make sure that we are practicing what we preach. This doesn't mean that we don't ever eat sugar or processed food. And it definitely doesn't mean that you can't ever eat a donut again. In our family, we simply try to eat the best we can at home and then when we are away enjoying a party or a vacation (or a donut!), we skip the guilt.

The food we eat and when and how we eat it is the foundation of health and one of the largest drivers behind optimizing performance. It ties in strongly with our stress, sleep, relationships and our ability to feel and live our purpose.

Food is such a massive topic—in fact, we already have another book started that is an in-depth look at what we should be eating to optimize our health and performance.

As we go over nutrition in this section, we'll touch briefly on what and when to eat and then focus on changing the way you think about homemade, healthy food. We'll talk about learning how to cook, how planning makes it easier, and how to make it fun.

We want to help you change your food culture. A better life awaits.

FINDING TRUTH

Science can offer a multitude of research for any side of an argument you want to present.

The butter versus margarine battle is one of the foremost examples of this. With news articles, magazine covers, and even dietary guidelines flip-flopping back and forth for the past sixty years, it's difficult for the average consumer to see past the fickle headlines to find evidence-based answers.

The trick is to do your homework and look a little deeper at the research. Who's funding it, who profits, how much did lobby groups with ties to Big Agra companies grant to the University that year?

Also, how well was it designed? How many people were involved in the study? Over what time period? What type of study was it? All these questions and more can give you a better idea of whether the research really can be trusted.

But at the bottom of it all, in a world of ever changing scientific evidence, we find a solid and sure base in scripture. We don't know everything about how to be healthy, and we won't in this lifetime. Luckily the One who made us and knows everything about how our bodies work and function optimally has provided some guidance in the form of scripture and speaking through prophets:

The Old Testament gives us direction in Daniel that a plant-based diet (seeds, grains, legumes, and vegetables) will bring greater health, strength, and knowledge than a diet of rich foods consisting primarily of meat and wine.

Ezra Taft Benson, who served part of his career as the U.S. Secretary of Agriculture before he became the president of the Church of Jesus Christ of Latter-day Saints stated,

> To a significant degree, we are an overfed and un-
> dernourished nation digging an early grave with our
> teeth, and lacking the energy that could be ours... We
> need a generation of young people who, as Daniel,
> eat in a healthier manner than to fare on the 'kings'
> meat'—and whose countenances show it.[61]

As members of the Church of Jesus Christ of Latter-day Saints, we have modern revelation that supports and expands on that. We are taught to eat meat sparingly, to have fruits and vegetables in abundance and in season, and to eat whole grains. We are directed to avoid strong drinks, including alcohol, coffee, and tea (from tea leaves, herbal tea is fine). We are also told to avoid tobacco and illegal drugs and taught to avoid any habit-forming and addictive substances.

Almost forty years ago, a UCLA researcher analyzed disease rates of 70,500 religiously active Mormon males in California and Utah. He found that they had 50% lower mortality rates from cancer than corresponding US white males of similar ages.[62]

An interesting thing to note is that our scriptural direction on health, called "The Word of Wisdom" begins with a warning to beware of conspiring minds. We have a pretty good idea of what that could mean.[63]

There are a lot of individuals, groups, and corporations which profit heavily from promoting products that line their pockets while harming our health. We need to be aware of that when reading articles and making food choices.

The Word of Wisdom states that it is adapted for the weakest of saints, or in other words, it is the lower law—the simple law. As we try to study and learn everything that modern science and ancient wisdom has to offer, we do it through the lens of this inspired revelation and seek our own personal revelation in pursuing a higher law as well. We also begin to understand the protective powers of following this health code as we see more and more disease.

Ezra Taft Benson also stated,

> There is no question that the health of the body affects the spirit, or the Lord would never have revealed the Word of Wisdom... Disease, fever and unexpected deaths are some of the consequences directly related to disobedience... To a great extent, we are physically what we eat. Most of us are acquainted with some of the prohibitions of the Word of Wisdom...but what need additional emphasis are the positive aspects— the need for vegetables, fruits, and grain, particularly wheat. We need a generation of people who eat in a healthier manner.[64]

When we understand that our nutrition affects our physical, mental, and spiritual health, then we also recognize that health-related commandments are meant to provide us blessings physical and spiritual.

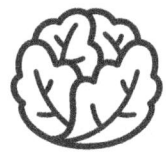

FOOD CULTURE

#1: Food Upgrade
Replace unhealthy food habits with clean eating habits.

#2: Cooking Class
Learn how to find joy in making healthy, real food

#3: Plan to Win
*Preparing ahead of time makes it easier
to make healthy meals.*

#4: Make Food Fun Again
*Celebrate good food! Plan activities, dates, and events
around healthy food.*

#5: Adjust Your Eating Schedule
When you eat is almost as important as what you eat.

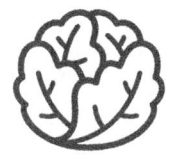

HABIT #1

FOOD UPGRADE

Replace unhealthy
food habits with
clean eating habits.

FOOD UPGRADE

It's really convenient to just grab something and go, but it's not at all convenient to deal with chronic disease. If you want to be at the top of your game mentally, physically, and emotionally, the best place to start is with your eating habits.

Fake foods fill up many kitchen pantries and, unfortunately, they cause more problems than they solve. Sometimes we just need a quick pick-me-up or something to calm the brewing hunger storm, but it only helps for a little while before we come crashing down again.

Sadly, many of us have a physiological and/or psychological addiction to these pseudo-foods. And it's not by accident—they have been engineered to be addictive.[9] Kelly Brownell, a Yale University professor of psychology and public health said,

> As a culture, we've become upset by the tobacco companies advertising to children, but we sit idly by while the food companies do the very same thing. And we could make a claim that the toll taken on the public health by a poor diet rivals that taken by tobacco.[10]

So how do you fight off the addiction and reclaim your freedom and energy?

1. Remove all food that isn't aligned with your goals.
When you are trying to get rid of bad habits, replacing is the key. If it's a habit to hit up the drive-through for a soda every afternoon, find something else to do instead. For example, keep coconut water, kombucha, or water kefir in your fridge or in a cooler in your car until you've broken the chain.

The temptation to eat bad food isn't as great if you don't actually have any in your house! Tell everyone you know so that friends and family can support you instead of innocently sabotaging your goals with supersized sodas and extra fries.

What in the world is actually in a can of cream of chicken soup? And have you been trying to pretend that the neon orange stuff in that mac and cheese box is even remotely related to actual cheese? Getting rid of processed and packaged food means banning the boxed cake mix, the cream of crap cans, the ramen noodles, and the sugar syrup cups with minimal fruit in them.

There are two ways to break up with bad food, based on your personality.

ALL OR NOTHING:
Go through your pantry with a trash bag and get rid of the junk. If you can take your stash to a local food pantry today, go for it. If not, it's more important to get it out of your house ASAP. Just toss it in the (outdoor) trash can where it belongs. Make up your mind and do it as fast as you can! Then immediately restock with healthy alternatives.

EASE INTO IT:
Make a commitment not to purchase unhealthy food anymore. Use up what you have and then replace it with healthier options.

Sometimes this method works better when you have children who are used to a certain way of eating. Some kids respond better if you can add in new recipes and foods a little at a time instead of cutting them off all at once.

REMOVE & REPLACE

SODA
Replace with sparkling water, water kefir, kombucha. Be sure to drink plenty of water. Be careful of "natural flavors"

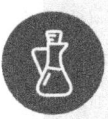

CANOLA/VEGETABLE OIL, MARGARINE, SHORTENING
Try avocado oil, coconut oil, olive oil, grass-fed butter or ghee, and animal fats (pastured lard, bacon fat, or grass-fed tallow).

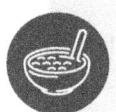

COLD CEREAL AND SUGAR OATMEAL PACKETS
Replace with steel-cut oats, granola sweetened with honey or fruit, muesli, soaked and baked whole grains.

CHIPS & CRACKERS
Switch for fresh cut veggies, raw nuts, olives, fermented vegetables, roasted seaweed, grass-fed beef jerky, and hard-boiled eggs.

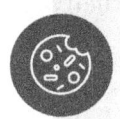

SWEET TREATS
Try fresh fruit, dates and other dried fruit, dried coconut, nut butters, energy balls, fat bombs, frozen almond milk pops. Sweeten homemade treats with honey, dates, pears, stevia, or monk fruit.

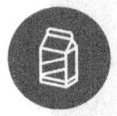

LOW-FAT OR REDUCED-FAT DAIRY
Use organic whole milk/full fat dairy, grass-fed and raw whenever possible, homemade nut or seed milk.

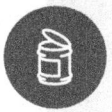

PROCESSED PACKAGED FOODS
Use fewer boxes and cans and eat more whole food, plant-based meals prepared at home.

2. Replace fake food habits with clean food habits.

As soon as the fake food is cleared out, you need to restock with healthy replacements. Costco offers many great organic and clean options, as well as most forward-thinking grocery stores. Some of our favorites are Trader Joe's, Whole Foods, Natural Grocers, Sprouts Farmers Market, and Wegmans. We also buy quite a bit online through various retailers and bulk group buy options.

If you recognize your weak spots (3 pm... every day) and are prepared with a replacement, then you can more easily fight the temptation when it strikes.

So, What to Eat?

This is the most frequently asked question in our office and in our home whenever we are having conversations about food.

For those that have been living the Standard American Diet (SAD), it's overwhelming to realize that most of what you have been filling your plate (or take-out container) with is probably not very good for you. Looking starvation in the face is intimidating!

We try to keep the focus positive and recognize all of the great things that you can eat. There is a learning curve for all knowledge worth gaining, and some people can ride it faster than others. Take it at your own pace.

The following chart shows the foods we believe to be part of an optimal eating plan (a modified Mediterranean diet) with a focus on eating local and seasonally as much as possible.

Fresh **Vegetables**

··

Fresh **Fruits**

··

Organic ancient **Whole Grains**, minimally processed and soaked as needed

··

Nuts and Seeds, soaked or sprouted as needed

··

Legumes, soaked as needed

··

Herbs and spices (for flavor and health benefits)

··

High-quality **Healthy Fats**

··

Wild-caught **Fish**

··

Raw grass-fed cultured **Dairy**, avoided in evenings and in winter (unless warmed with spices)

··

Organic homemade **Bone Broth**

··

Organic and humanely raised **Meat** with organs and bones, predominantly in winter and always in moderation.

Jar by Andres Ruales from the Noun Project

It's important to note that we frequently prescribe specific diets for patients, including a temporary elimination diet, anti-inflammatory diets, a paleo diet, a phytonutrient diet, a cyclical keto diet, the GAPS (gut-healing) diet, an auto-immune protocol, a hormone balancing diet, etc.

Some of these prescribed diets may be long-term eating plans, but most are intended to heal the body to be able to eat a broader range of food, as clean and close to nature as possible.

Fake Food

There are a few things that are conspicuously missing from the table, but if you can cut them out of your kitchen, you won't miss the way they sap your energy, your brainpower, and your health!

Why do we refer to these foods as fake? In contrast to the nutrient rich, antioxidant, anti-inflammatory, and health-promoting foods listed on the previous page, fake foods have their genesis in a lab instead of the earth.

Not only does fake food lack the health benefits of real food, many can have a detrimental effect on health.[11] Our bodies are miraculous machines and I've been amazed at how some can endure despite being fueled with suboptimal nutrition for years. However, the ill effects of poor nutrition inevitably manifest—and it's not pretty.

TIP: When grocery shopping, skip the middle of the store and just walk around the outside edges. You'll pass over almost all of the packaged foods. Utilize the bulk section for nuts, seeds, and grains.

Here's our list of things to avoid if you're trying to optimize your health and performance:

PROCESSED FOODS
Packaged, boxed, and
preservative-laden foods

....

PROCESSED SUGARS AND ARTIFICIAL SWEETENERS
White refined sugar, high fructose corn syrup,
aspartame, sucralose.

....

STIMULANTS
Remove all caffeine and alcohol from your home.
If you choose to drink, do so only in social situations
and sparingly.

....

HIGHLY PROCESSED FATS AND OILS
Vegetable oil, canola oil, Crisco, margarine.

....

GMO FOODS
Many crops (including corn, soy, canola, alfalfa,
cotton, and sorghum) are genetically modified to be
resistant to pesticides and herbicides so that farmers
can spray fields to kill weeds without killing their
crops. Those weed killers stay on (and inside) your
food, disrupting your hormones[65] and genes.[66] Toxins
can negatively impact your performance and overall
health, and for some of our patients, completely
compromise it.

ABOUT 5 MINUTES into our 60-minute visit, Shawn[12] began describing how he had been battling ADHD since first grade.

He began taking Ritalin when he was twenty-four, then shifted to Adderall and thought it was the best thing that ever happened to him. He was shocked at the ability it gave him to concentrate for hours and he became much more productive at work.

It didn't take long for Shawn to realize that if he took twice the recommended dose he felt even better.

As happens far too often, he soon found himself obsessed with and completely dependent on the medication. Shawn started to get tangled in the stronghold of addiction and deceit, trying to hide the evidence from his wife, and making questionable decisions.

Shawn started seeking out prescriptions from multiple doctors. He began sacrificing important things in his life in order to make sure he got enough of the drug, causing a major strain on his marriage and bringing him to the brink of divorce.

As we discussed Shawn's life—his sleep habits, nutrition, and stress management—and reviewed his advanced lab panel results, it became apparent that there were several contributing factors that he could start working on to improve his attention and focus.

As we discussed some of these underlying causes of Shawn's attention deficit disorder and addictive behavior, his posture shifted. As he recognized that this diagnosis wasn't "just him," but something that he could control, everything changed for him.

When Shawn realized that there were sustainable ways to improve his concentration and maintain his productivity at work, his entire outlook changed.

He felt hopeful and empowered, and motivated to fix and strengthen his relationship with his wife, Beth, and to be a better father to their three young children.

As is often the case, we began with the basics:

1. We removed inflammatory foods from his diet. *Note: Some top inflammatory foods are sugar, high fructose corn syrup, hydrogenated oils, vegetable oil, refined carbs/processed foods, processed meat, and alcohol.*

2. We upped his intake of vegetables (including fermented vegetables like sauerkraut, kimchi, and pickles) to provide critical vitamins and nutrients and improve his gut health.

3. We increased healthy fats, as his cholesterol was quite low, including the beneficial HDL.

4. We discussed personalized stress management techniques. Specifically, spending time outside in nature and grounding/earthing (direct physical connection with the earth.)

Shawn and Beth opted to do everything together with these nutrition and lifestyle changes.

They started making meals together and cooking became a fun and productive new hobby that also helped strengthen their relationship. They made a goal to take walks together each morning.

Shawn and Beth both noticed immediate improvement. Shawn couldn't wait to leave the drug and his previous struggles behind. Although we had decided together to slowly wean off of the Adderall, within two weeks Shawn opted to stop the medication altogether.[13]

As Shawn's natural ability to concentrate returned, he noticed that it didn't feel the same as the medication-induced focus. He was able to focus for longer amounts of time. He also started noticing how different foods made him feel and realized he was craving fish, avocados, nuts, seeds, healthy oils, and was even starting to crave fermented foods. All of these, of course, were exactly the foods that his body needed to heal itself and replenish the deficiencies he had.

The end result was a drastic and sustainable improvement in both Shawn's overall health and in Shawn and Beth's marriage. Their new-found hobbies and motivation to work together brought trust, friendship, and excitement into their relationship.

In general, the more food we eat in its natural state and the less it is refined without additives, the healthier it will be for us.[67]

EZRA TAFT BENSON

Why Good Food Matters

Does it really matter what food we eat? How we prepare and cook food? Whether the food was doused in pesticides or grown organically?[14] Whether the seeds were GMO?[15] Whether the animals were crowded into small plots of mud and feces, fed antibiotic-laden (and often pesticide-heavy, genetically modified[16]) soy or raised on open farmland, grazing on grass?

We all know people who live on fast food, junk food, and packaged food most of their lives and seem to get along just fine, right? That's just it though. Is our goal to get along just fine, knowing that what we are eating isn't ideal, but hoping it never catches up to us? Or, is our goal to thrive?

Couples who are seeking to optimize their performance in every aspect of their lives shouldn't settle for eating the food that is making major food and beverage companies wealthy and the world over-weight, fatigued, foggy, less productive, and full of digestive woes.

No. Our goal is to rise above the marketing tricks, the social norms, the easy and convenient ways, and to be able to reach our true potential.

So, YES, it really does matter what we eat. The type of food we eat, along with how it is grown, harvested, prepared, and cooked all matters. This may seem extreme to some, but it's really just common sense—with medical research to back it up.

Nutrition Research

Brand new research out of Loma Linda University links an unhealthy diet to mental illness in California adults[17]—backing up previous studies with similar findings. For example, having a sweet tooth has been found to be associated with bipolar disorder and eating a lot of fried foods, processed grains, and sugar has been linked to depression.[18]

ORGANIC VS. CONVENTIONALLY GROWN

A study published in the *Public Health Nutrition Journal* in 2017 looked at how eating organic food during pregnancy was associated with different health-related markers. They tested 1339 pregnant women and found that consumption of organic food was associated with a more favorable pre-pregnancy BMI (height to weight ratio) and lower prevalence of gestational diabetes.[19]

There are many studies showing decreased occurrence of allergies, asthma, and eczema in families with a diet that includes organic food.[20,21,22,23,24,25]

Research done in the Netherlands followed 2700 pregnant women and their children. The children whose mothers consumed organic dairy products when pregnant and who themselves were given organic dairy after weaning had a 36% reduction in the risk of eczema at the age of two years old versus the children who had conventional non-organic dairy exposure in-utero and after birth.[26]

Perhaps the first ever prospective study investigating weight change over time related to intake of organic food was called the NutriNet-Santé study and included 62,000 participants.[27,28] BMI increase and risk of obesity over time were both lower among high consumers of organic food compared to low consumers.

The NutriNet-Santé study also showed that organic food consumers (occasional and regular), as compared to non-consumers, exhibited a lower incidence of hypertension, type 2 diabetes, high cholesterol levels (both men and women), and cardiovascular disease (men only).[29]

TOXIC FOOD PACKAGING

Not only do we need to be aware of and educate ourselves about the safety of the food we eat; we also need to consider how it is packaged. Chemicals commonly used in food packaging "…have been associated with endocrine disruption in animals and in some human studies."

When these chemicals build up in our bodies, they can contribute to many different health issues.

How often do you drink from a can? A study published in *Hypertension Journal* concluded that drinking from cans increases your blood pressure.[30]

The good news is, our bodies are built to detox. When our systems are working efficiently it doesn't take long to show a marked drop in toxins once we stop the exposure.

A study where participants switched to an organic, fresh food diet with no cans or plastic packaging showed that it only took a few days for measurable levels of industrial chemicals used in plastics to drop significantly. BPA levels detected in the body decreased by 66% and phthalate levels dropped by over 50% within just three days.[31]

The easiest way to decrease the problems (and packaging!) that occur before the food gets to our tables and tummies is to decrease the journey. The shorter the trip between the farm and the table, the more likely we are to have safe, nutrient-dense, and good-tasting food.

Fresh + Local

While growing up, we both had the awesome opportunity to spend summer and fall eating from gardens and orchards. Scott was raised on a cherry orchard and Amy grew up in Fruit Heights... which—you guessed it—was also full of orchards, including her parent's backyard orchard full of fruit trees of every kind.

Our parents saw the value in growing a garden and we were raised to enjoy bright red tomatoes fresh off the vine, golden corn husked right before dinner, and an endless rotation of in-season fruit.

No grocery store tomato can ever quite compare with what you'll find in a backyard garden or at the farmer's market. And we don't even bother buying cherries from a store most of the time.

Why does home-grown, local food taste so much better?

Local produce is grown primarily for taste. Grocery store produce is bred for appearance, high yield, disease resistance, and an ability to travel—taste is often sacrificed.

God created food that would taste the best when its nutritional value was fully optimized. When we pick fruit before it is ripe, not only does it not taste as good, but the nutrition isn't as developed as it could be.

For example, one of the health-promoting properties found in blackberries is four times higher when they are completely ripe.[32]

Much of the fruit you'll find at the store was picked underdeveloped and hard so that it could travel well and then force-ripened with ethylene gas. Lengthy shipping time and suboptimal storing temperatures also degrade nutrient values of produce.[33]

Home gardens are grown in small plots and rotated more frequently, meaning the soil isn't depleted by mono-cropping. Homegrown produce has access to more nutrients and minerals than most supermarket produce.

In the garden, the better the food is for you, the better it tastes. Nothing can compare in taste, texture, and variety to fresh, healthy food that is skillfully prepared.

If enjoying the taste of healthy food hasn't been your experience it is because you haven't had the chance to see how good healthy food can really be. It's probably because in the past you have equated healthy food with overcooked vegetables with no seasoning and meals devoid of fat and salt... two very important things for our bodies and two VERY important things for taste.

The best tasting and the healthiest meals are born in a backyard garden or a local farm.[34] The best restaurants you'll eat at will be sourcing their produce, meat, and dairy locally. Their chefs will have been up early that morning, fighting over the produce picked the night before and driven into the city at 4 am. They will go back and make their own sauces, clean and chop their own veggies, and create most of their masterpieces from fresh food, not canned.

You deserve to eat this way all the time but, unless you have an unlimited food budget, you're going to need to learn to make your own masterpieces. Embrace fresh and local and you'll be most of the way there!

Replace unhealthy food habits
with clean eating habits.

NEW HABIT FORMATION

Write down the habit you would like to incorporate, including when you will do it. Whenever possible, pair the desired habit with an existing habit. For situational habits designate an if...then clause.

EXAMPLES

- Pack a lunch each morning after breakfast instead of grabbing something on-the-go.

- We'll pack a cooler in our car with coconut water so that IF we get a drive-thru soda craving, THEN we have a better option.

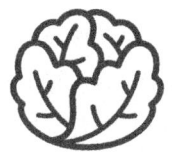

HABIT #2

C O O K I N G
C L A S S

Learn how to find joy in making healthy, real food

COOKING CLASS

We love our Saturday morning trips to the Farmer's Market. It's become a weekly ritual to bring home baskets full of freshly picked produce and artisan raw milk cheese, (along with the occasional keto cupcake!) It's fun to get ideas from the farmers about how to prepare food in new ways and we love to look up recipes online to creatively use our new ingredients.

A *Business Insider* article from 2017 referencing US Bureau of Labor Statistics reported that Americans spend most of their food budget on pre-made food. The three largest food expenditures are eating out, miscellaneous foods, and nonalcoholic beverages—and they make up 60% of average annual household spending on food![35]

Not knowing how to cook and prepare real food is one of the biggest roadblocks to good nutrition. Dedicate yourself to learning how to cook healthy food as though it's your new profession.

If you can set aside two meals a week to experiment with an exciting new whole food recipe, by the end of the month you'll have eight healthy recipes under your belt. That's amazing progress!

One of our favorite places to find inspiration is Pinterest (we all know that pictures sell food!) Enter search terms like:

- Clean eating recipes
- Whole food, plant-based recipes
- AIP (Auto-Immune Protocol) recipes
- Whole30 recipes
- Paleo recipes
- Keto recipes
- Weston Price or WAPF (Weston A. Price Foundation) recipes

Not knowing
how to prepare
and cook real food
is one of the biggest
roadblocks to
good nutrition.

To be clear, we don't advocate paleo or keto diets for everyone, but searching for recipes under those terms will weed out recipes with sugar and white flour. This will provide you with some excellent options to include in your personalized nutrition plan, as recommended by your doctor, based on your lab results and genetic testing.

TIP: If your doctor doesn't order or review advanced labs (including micronutrients, microbiome, hormones, allergies, genetics, and toxins), seek out a doctor who has done additional training in functional medicine. IFM.org is a great resource for finding trained practitioners in your area if you prefer having a local physician.

You can also search for blogs or cookbooks with similar search terms. There's an endless number of free healthy recipes available online, but if you love to hold them in your hands (total cookbook junkies here…we're with you), there are loads of amazing cookbooks filled with healthy recipes that will keep you full and satisfied longer than a microwave dinner could ever dream of.

So, create a DIY cooking class. Sit down together one evening and find some recipes that make your mouth water and get you excited about this new team sport called cooking. Maybe it's a new main dish for Friday night and a great brunch recipe for Sunday morning.

The hardest part might honestly be limiting it to two new recipes. If you want to make more than that, don't worry, we won't tell anybody.

The fundamental attributes that you will need are a willingness to learn together, a desire to experiment with cooking and eating new things, and the assumption that you can fail together and laugh about it. Yes, that happens sometimes! (We're thinking of Scott's overnight key lime chia seed pudding [disgusting!] and his sister Sharon's coconut flour pancakes which reportedly turned into scramble.)

Commit to an environment with no criticism, only laughter. Creativity and experimentation make everything more fun.

Make a cultural shift to embrace and eat real food. Visit farmers markets together on Saturday mornings. Join a food share or co-op, visit local farms, and go pick fruit at the orchard together. Embrace how real food changes with the seasons.

As you discover your new talent for cooking (and even better—a new love of eating clean!) your whole mindset around food will change. You'll feel empowered and excited about healthy food.

"It is an exceedingly difficult thing for most people to break off and discontinue cherished and long-standing habits...We can have variety in diet, and yet have simplicity. We can have a diet that will be easily prepared, and yet have it healthful. We can have a diet that will be tasteful, nutritious and delightful to us and easy to digest..." [68]

GEORGE Q. CANNON

Learn how to find joy in making healthy, real food

NEW HABIT FORMATION

Write down the habit you would like to incorporate, including when you will do it. Whenever possible, pair the desired habit with an existing habit. For situational habits designate an if...then clause.

EXAMPLES

- Before heading to the farmer's market and grocery store on Saturdays, look up a new recipe to try for Sunday dinner.

- Start a Pinterest board for healthy snacks or treats; choose one recipe to make each Monday afternoon and keep the extras in the freezer for spur-of-the-moment needs.

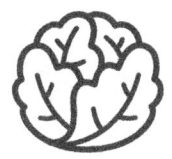

HABIT #3

PLAN
TO WIN

Preparing ahead of time makes it easier to make healthy meals.

PLAN TO WIN

Our scriptures teach that "if ye are prepared ye shall not fear."[36]

If you think of fear in the context of anxiousness (a very common form of fear), then this can be a valuable admonition for food preparation. If you plan ahead and prepare before it's time to actually make the meal then you skip the anxiety of realizing it's somehow already 6 pm, the kids are fighting, everybody is suddenly starving, and you have no idea what to cook.

Planning minimizes stress and leads to success.

With the previous challenge to find new recipes to try each week, you're already on your way to developing a solid meal plan.

The next step is to set aside a time each week for meal prep (doing some of the work ahead of time.) This might include cleaning and chopping all the veggies for the next few meals in one night. It might mean that you start your breakfast the night before so that it's easy to finish up first thing in the morning.

Meal prep is a great boon for couples who work and aren't left with as much time for cooking. It's also great for couples with children at home that seem to require all your attention as soon as you're trying to cook a meal.

If you feel like you don't have a lot of time to prepare meals each day, designate one day a week as meal prep day and spend 30-60 minutes meal prepping for the rest of the week. The most convenient times for most of our patients seem to be Saturday afternoons after grocery shopping or one evening a week after the kids go to bed.

Some examples of things that you can do ahead of time are:

- Chop vegetables and fruit
- Start homemade bone broth to cook overnight
- Make dressings or sauces
- Roast vegetables and proteins that can be used for multiple meals
- Assemble salad jars
- Mix up sourdough waffles or bread to bake the next day
- Start overnight oats or chia seed pudding before heading to bed
- Or here's an easy one: just plan to double one or two meals each week and refrigerate or freeze the extra meal for later.

While some couples really enjoy doing meal prep together and utilize the "busy work" as a great time to talk, it's also a wonderful thing to do together as a family. There's research to suggest that involving your kids in meal prep helps them maintain a better diet through young adulthood.[37]

In fact, another study shows that the number of home-prepared, family meals in a household can be predicted by the number of food preparation supplies and equipment available in that house.[38] So, if your goal is to have more home-prepared family meals (and we're hoping it is!), then think about allocating a little bit of your budget to invest in some high-quality food prepping supplies.

Some food prep tools that we use weekly—if not daily—are:

HIGH-POWERED BLENDER
- To make nut milk, sauces, and smoothies
- To blend up pancake or waffle batter

FOOD PROCESSOR
- To make nut butters, salsas, fillings, pesto's, and pastry dough
- To grate cheese and veggies

IMMERSION BLENDER
- To make homemade mayo, aioli, and salad dressing
- To puree soups and sauces
- To blend baby food

ELECTRIC MIXER
- To mix baked goods, knead bread, or quickly mix up eggs.
- We also have a spiralizer attachment that we use to make zucchini, squash, beet, and sweet potato noodles.

DEHYDRATOR
- To dehydrate sprouted almonds and soaked nuts/seeds
- To dehydrate sprouted grains
- To dehydrate fruit
- To make crackers

Oh, and let's just throw it out there that a good set of knives is going to be your favorite thing when you are meal prepping.

No kidding, we often take our knives with us when we go on road trips or to visit family. It is not fun (or very safe) to try to cut food quickly with a cheap, dull knife. We've even been known to gift knives to loved ones so that we can use them when we go to their house. (We're not always selfish gift givers, just when it comes to meal prep!)

When you have a plan and the resources you need, all of a sudden everything seems a lot easier and you realize you can do it!

BEN, A HARDWORKING 35-year-old father of four girls, was having chronic headaches which were becoming unbearable. The headaches started a few years before but were mild and intermittent until the past few months, when they had become debilitating.

By the time I saw Ben, he rarely had days without headaches and would sometimes have to leave work to go home and sleep—which was the only way he could find relief.

Multiple visits with Ben's primary care doctor and specialists hadn't provided an answer. He'd had an MRI and other testing—none of which revealed any abnormalities. He was told that the headaches were caused by stress and was offered heavy medications. Wisely, he rejected the medications and continued to seek other solutions.

Ben's previous job required a lot of time away from his family and was extremely stressful. For these reasons, he left that job 6 months earlier, effectively eliminating most of the stress in his life. His headaches were increasing despite this healthy career transition, indicating that these were not stress-induced episodes.

Exercise and heavy exertion seemed to make Ben's headaches worse. Where he was previously running, lifting weights, and doing other exercise daily, he was now barely able to tolerate his daily activities at work.

Other symptoms which afflicted Ben included fatigue, indigestion and other gut issues, lack of clarity, and trouble concentrating.

I was initially concerned that Ben's headaches might be due to exposure to toxins and high voltage power lines because he had been working around chemicals and power lines for several years. However, after getting back his lab work and seeing a few nutrient deficiencies and blood sugar imbalances, we decided to start with a change in nutrition and add some professional-grade supplements.

Although they were both busy in their careers and with their young family, Ben and Heather were highly motivated to find a solution to his headaches and jumped right into a strict elimination diet. They removed all potential allergens and food triggers from their diet for several weeks before slowly adding them back in one at a time while tracking symptoms.

As is the case for almost everybody, there were some major initial changes which had to be made, including adding in a lot more vegetables and healthy fats, as well as removing soda and processed, packaged foods with corn, soy, sugar, or other preservatives. Although it was difficult, they both began to see beneficial effects within the first week.

Within several weeks, both Ben and Heather were losing weight, feeling more energized and looking healthier. Ben previously had a lot inflammation throughout his body, and it was interesting how quickly the redness and puffiness in his face diminished. He had a few headaches the first few days as part of the initial detox but has since been headache free.

One of the other great benefits to this lifestyle shift was to hear Ben and Heather talk about how planning, shopping, and making food together strengthened their relationship. Having a united goal and purpose, the opportunity to work together in learning new skills, and enjoying the fruits of their labors brought a new dimension to their relationship.

We have seen this time and again—when a couple works together to alter their lifestyle, it brings them closer and creates a sustainable change. Accountability is huge in any change or progression, and having a partner makes all the difference.

We have many patients who succeed on their own as well, and sometimes despite having an unsupportive spouse. But it is sad when a couple misses out on an opportunity to strengthen their life together. Working together builds momentum and excitement that is hard to find elsewhere.

Our personal and business mission statements both include the verbiage that we exist to support and build healthy families. Our ideal clients are a husband and wife who are united in their vision for a healthy and happy life and are willing to work together to learn how to achieve those goals.

When only one spouse is willing to make lifestyle changes, it tends to invite resentment and increase stress. Since stress induces detrimental change in gut bacteria and a host of other health implications, this is completely counterproductive to our mission.

Preparing ahead of time makes it easier to make healthy meals.

NEW HABIT FORMATION

Write down the habit you would like to incorporate, including when you will do it. Whenever possible, pair the desired habit with an existing habit. For situational habits designate an if...then clause.

EXAMPLES

- On Sundays after our walk we will make five jars of overnight oats so that we can pull one out each weekday morning and have breakfast ready in minutes.

- Right after grocery shopping, we will chop up veggies for the week.

_____

_____

_____

_____

_____

_____

_____

_____

_____

_____

_____

_____

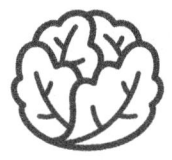

HABIT #4

MAKE HEALTHY FUN

Celebrate good food! Plan activities, dates, and events around healthy food.

MAKE HEALTHY FUN

When you hear the word "healthy" what comes to mind? Do you think cardboard crackers or your grandma's bran muffins? Bland green beans or mushy brussels sprouts?

Or do you think of juicy just-picked orchard peaches, crisp bell peppers, or mouth-watering fresh-caught Alaskan salmon?

The better your mindset around food, the better your nutrition and health outcomes will be. If your experience with "healthy" food is negative, you're going to need to trust us on this one until you find out for yourself: Real food, well prepared, can (and will) be the best food you've ever eaten. And eating the best food can be so much fun!

And it's not just eating—cooking doesn't feel like so much work anymore when you're having fun with it! For us, the key to having fun cooking is to do it together.

Build your food culture by inviting friends over to cook with you or to share a meal that you make. Find new healthy farm-to-table restaurants. Experiment with making food from other countries and cultures.

This is a big one: replace all negative thoughts and talk regarding food. Phrases such as, "I am not a good cook," or "I don't like to bake," or "I don't like to eat onions." Be adventurous and try new things with people that you love.

Eating with Friends
The joy of eating together and making meals for and eating with other families can break down barriers and build new bonds.

Inviting other families over for meals is a tradition started by Amy's parents and has been one of the greatest blessings in our lives. This has been the single best way for us (and our kids) to make friends.

We've always made friends quickly whenever we have moved (and we've moved a lot—ten times in our fifteen years of marriage) because we're willing to bribe people with food to be our friends. Some meals have been better than others, but most people are willing to overlook experimental meals and still want to be friends even if we serve them raw chicken (yep, done that), or chili so spicy that it makes grown men cry (done that too.)

Food is the basis of a lot of our friendships—and many of our best memories! Hannah and Jason were some of our first food friends. Our next-door neighbors in student housing, they knew us when we were just learning to love cooking and stuck with us through many experimental dinners.

One of our favorite memories is sitting outside of a campground bathroom with Jason and Hannah playing card games while our homemade ice cream churned inside, utilizing the only power outlet for miles. You could probably hear it for miles too…the middle of the desert is a quiet place at night! Later on, when they talked us into moving to Hawaii with them for a few months, we made many more food memories and gained an undying love of seafood.

Not only did we make friends by cooking and eating with them, we also made friends by watching cooking shows with them. Back in our college days, our friends Jordan and Shayna co-hosted Iron Chef parties with us on Sunday nights. One of us would invite a new couple each week and we got to know a lot of people and a lot of new cooking techniques at the same time.

We have learned that the more that you know about cooking food, the less intimidating it is to try new recipes and figure out how to make things in a healthier way.

Food can help you make new friends, and food can also cement the friendships that you have. Sharing food experiences together creates strong memories because you're engaging all of your senses. Memories are based on sensory experience. "The same part of the brain that's in charge of processing our senses is also responsible, at least in part, for storing emotional memories."[39]

For many years, when we would travel back home for a summer vacation or Christmas break, we would gather with some of our best friends from home and everybody would share something delicious.

Talesha and Clint made us colorfully complex food and empowered us to feel confident trying our hand at making it ourselves. We still remember the silky texture of Heather's pots de crème and walking into the house to find the amazing smell of Shayne's Saturday morning breakfast.

These traditions and memories make up our passion for food, which in turn fuels our passion for health and nutrition. If you can start to experience healthy food in a new way, with all your senses and with people you love, then your association becomes positive and your mindset shifts to empower you to greater health.

Cooking with Kids

It's really helpful to involve your children as you develop new attitudes towards food and cooking. If they see you having fun in the kitchen together, they want to be there with you! Teaching your children to enjoy making food will help them for the rest of their lives.

Let them do "big" things. Teach them how to use a knife safely. Let them crack eggs and measure. They soak up the responsibility and can learn many skills that they might otherwise miss out on.

Make your family meal times an event to look forward to. Let the kids be in charge of choosing recipes for one meal a week. Designate themed food nights. Make Taco Tuesday a thing in your house.

There are so[40] many[41] studies[42] showing[43] that[44] families[45] who eat meals together have healthier children, physically and emotionally.

Make It Special

Celebrate holidays with special food. Research Irish recipes for St. Paddy's or give it a green theme. Make heart pancakes for Valentine's Day. Pumpkin spice everything for the month of October.

We loved living in Chicago, but there is no denying that the winters can be long and dark. Some of our favorite people, Burke and Salem, helped us make it through by celebrating holidays the same way we do… with ALL the food. Sometimes, we made up our own holidays just so that we could experiment with more great recipes.

Discovering obscure holidays builds endless food excitement. If you can name it, there's probably a holiday for it. Go live it up and start celebrating National Turkey Neck Soup Day[46]… because, why not?

A few of our favorite food traditions are centered around birthdays and Christmas. For birthdays, the kids get to decide everything that we make and eat the whole day. There is yearlong planning that goes into these birthday menus—and frequent changes until the last possible minute. Just yesterday, our seven-year-old (whose birthday is not for four more months) informed us of his updated menu. Our friend,

Bruce, makes birthdays special for his wife Melinda in the same way. Each year we look forward to hearing the celebration menu!

For the past few years, we've embraced a new tradition of researching a different country's Christmas traditions and recipes, culminating in a special Christmas Eve dinner. This past year we celebrated Iceland. The dinner menu consisted of baked wild-caught salmon and smashed potatoes with a creamy cashew yogurt dill sauce, red cabbage and onion slaw, Scott's homemade sourdough bread, and a citrus arugula salad. But the thing our kids keep talking about is the blueberry skyr (Icelandic yogurt) tarts we made for dessert.

Our good friends, Brandon and Lana Lewis, are great examples of getting their kids excited about food. Every week they pick a country or culture to learn about during the week and then cook their traditional foods on Saturday.

Making mealtimes meaningful has so many benefits and results in healthier food and healthier relationships.

Don't Let Tech Get in The Way

It's important to make meals a distraction-free zone. Some families ban phones from the dinner table. It's well documented that watching TV while eating is associated with weight gain[47] and a lower quality diet.[48]

Basically, your mind and your body need to be on the same page for your digestion to work optimally. If your brain doesn't realize you are eating because you are completely consumed by your new favorite series, then your brain won't signal that you are full. You miss out on all the satisfaction of eating and end up consuming more than you usually would and should.

Celebrate good food! Plan activities, dates, and events around healthy food.

NEW HABIT FORMATION

Write down the habit you would like to incorporate, including when you will do it. Whenever possible, pair the desired habit with an existing habit. For situational habits designate an if...then clause.

EXAMPLES

- We will find somebody at church each week to invite to dinner the following Friday night —at our house or at a healthy restaurant.

- We'll plan a food culture night once a month and invite friends to join in.

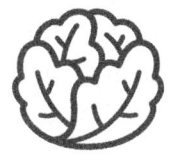

HABIT #5

ADJUST YOUR EATING SCHEDULE

When you eat is almost as important as what you eat.

ADJUST YOUR EATING SCHEDULE

For many people with fast moving lifestyles, a good breakfast and lunch are a luxury and dinner is their only real meal. Thus, many busy professionals find themselves eating most of their food at a late hour after a long day of work.

This late-night eating schedule invites some big problems into your life; problems such as a higher risk for obesity, diabetes, and the C-word.

A published review of several human intervention trials summarized that "eating the majority of calories later in the day may be detrimental for glycemic control." [49]

Another study stated that "Compared with subjects sleeping immediately after supper, those sleeping two or more hours after supper had a 20% reduction in cancer risk for breast and prostate cancer combined." [50]

In a world where almost 40% of us will have cancer[51], is lowering your cancer risk by 20% good enough to motivate you to shift your schedule?

The goal is to fuel up your body when it is actively converting energy (during the day) and then eat easy-to-digest foods in the evening. This will allow your body to focus more energy on healing the gut and detoxing the brain.

New research is showing that some people become more insulin resistant at the end of the day, making it even more advantageous for them to move their eating schedule forward.[52]

So, make breakfast and lunch (or brunch and supper) your main meals. Go big and you shouldn't be nearly as prone to snacking between meals. Amy's dad made a great tradition of eating well first thing. He was in the kitchen first thing, making a hot, hearty breakfast for their family every morning before school.

If, after a big breakfast and lunch, you are still hungry in the evening, drink water or some hot herbal tea. If you're still hungry thirty minutes later, eat something light, such as soup or salad, vegetables or fruit. As a general rule, avoid meat, bread, dairy, and sugar after 5 pm as many times a week as you can. If that's hard for you, start with twice a week and work up from there.

Circadian Rhythm and Eating

The timing and consistent scheduling of your meals also plays into your body's circadian rhythms. We talk a lot more about this in the sleep section, but maintaining optimal circadian rhythm plays a massive role in your overall health.

Research demonstrates the effect that mealtimes can have on standardizing circadian rhythms and shows that selectively adjusting meal times can benefit shift workers and frequent travelers.[53]

Do you travel for work? How about deadlines at work that require some late nights? Keeping your standard mealtimes might help you bounce back a lot faster!

Data from one study suggests that being intentional about when you eat "could lead to a healthier lifestyle and cardiometabolic risk factor management." [54]

Allowing your body a prolonged amount of time without eating, is called fasting. More and more studies are showing that intermittent fasting has many benefits.[55] One method is to fast one to two days a week. Our preferred method of intermittent fasting is to limit eating to certain hours each day.

A supervised controlled trial by University of Alabama researchers, showed that restricting the eating window to six hours a day (with dinner before 3 pm, to coincide with circadian rhythms) improved blood pressure, oxidative stress, insulin sensitivity, and appetite.[56]

The benefits of intermittent fasting for weight loss and metabolism are well-supported. Dr. Deborah Wexler, director of the Mass General Hospital Diabetes Center and associate professor at Harvard Medical School is quoted in a *Harvard Health* article saying, "There is evidence to suggest that the circadian rhythm fasting approach, where meals are restricted to an eight to ten-hour period of the daytime, is effective." [57]

An NPR report shared the following research notes in favor of eating earlier:

> "...people who ate their main meal earlier in the day were much more successful at losing weight," says study author Frank Scheer, a Harvard neuroscientist who directs the Medical Chronobiology Program at Brigham and Women's Hospital. In fact, early eaters lost 25 percent more weight than later eaters — 'a surprisingly large difference,' Scheer says.[58]

Another study found that eating a big breakfast was more conducive to weight loss, compared with a big dinner—adding to the evidence that the timing of meals is important.[59]

We fast for 24 hours the first Sunday of each month as part of our religious observance. It's interesting to see the benefits of just a once-a-month fast published in a study based on 448 hospital patients. "[Participants] who reported routine fasting (29%) exhibited significantly lower weight and lower fasting glucose levels, as well as lower prevalences of diabetes and coronary stenosis." [60]

Real Life Though

So, what does this concept look like for a family? It can be adapted to different needs, but for us it means eating a hearty morning meal around 7 am and our main meal around 3 pm at least 3-4 days a week.

Breakfast is an area where meal prep can really pay off. We mix up chia seed pudding and sourdough pancakes, segment grapefruit and chop veggies for omelets, or start some overnight before bed so that we are ready to roll the next morning. Eggs are also frequent fliers at our breakfast table. Scrambled eggs, fried eggs, soft boiled, hard boiled, and baked eggs somehow all feel different enough that the kids don't complain that they're eating the same thing all the time.

Scott scheduled his lunch for early afternoon so that he can often run home and eat with us. Two of our kids don't arrive home from school until 3:30, so they pack their own lunch and then we keep dinner warm for them or reheat.

We'll often have leftover soup, salad, or a smoothie all together around 6 pm, but sometimes we are satisfied to just have some hot ginger, lemon, & honey tea and call it a night.

Our kids are noticeably calmer and happier when we eat earlier. If they are eating well enough during meals, we let them snack on fruit, veggies, or nuts if they get hungry between meals.

One immediate benefit is that the dreaded dinner hour has vanished. This shift has removed all of the stress and expectations of having a big dinner on the table every night. The kids don't get hangry, because they can eat a real meal right when they walk in the door from school. Rather than busily making dinner when our children are finally home, we can be completely present while they are showing-off their school projects or when they need help with homework.

When we follow this schedule and eat early our evenings are much more likely to be happy and smooth. When we don't, those hours between school and dinner revert right back to what many parents not-so-affectionately refer to as the hardest part of the day.

Another benefit to eating earlier is the way we feel about sleep. When we do eat late (usually in social situations), we want to push back bedtime because we feel too full to go to sleep. But when we stay on schedule, we feel great when we go to bed, sleep much better, and wake up more refreshed.

Some couples meet for lunch during the day and bring home leftovers for kids to eat when they arrive home from school. Some couples spend Sunday evenings preparing and packing great lunches to take to work during the week.

Look at your life and see how it will work out for you to shift things. Even if you can only do it a few days a week, you'll still see benefits! We have made it a rule that doing a little better each day is always a win. This is not an all or nothing sort of game!

FOOD & SPIRITUALITY

Personal experience has taught us that we are able to be much more spiritually in-tune when our bodies are not weighed down with excessive food, unhealthy foods, or any type of stimulant.

Recognizing spiritual promptings requires a clear mind. Have you ever experienced a "food coma"? Or desperately needed a siesta? When we eat too much (even if it is good food!) an excessive amount of energy is diverted to digestion, robbing the body of the ability to utilize energy for any higher purposes.

Along with not eating too much, we also want to make sure that we eat enough. Eating enough is really more about quality than quantity, though. We need enough high-quality food to get all of the essentials for good physical and mental health.

Rewind a few years to your high school psychology classes and bring Maslow's hierarchy of needs back to mind. Maslow wrote in 1943 in "A Theory of Human Motivation"[69] that man must fulfill basic physical needs before spiritual awareness or enlightenment is achieved.

We live this truth daily. We need to allow our bodies and minds the ability to surpass the physical needs in order to attain spirituality.

If we are always digesting (because we are frequently eating or snacking), then we can't ever get beyond physical mode. This leaves no energy or time preserved for spiritual nourishment.

When you eat is almost as important as what you eat.

NEW HABIT FORMATION

Write down the habit you would like to incorporate, including when you will do it. Whenever possible, pair the desired habit with an existing habit. For situational habits designate an if...then clause.

EXAMPLES

- We'll eat dinner at 5 pm and not eat anything after 6 pm. IF we feel hungry in the evening, THEN we will drink some warm herbal tea.

- We'll do a 24-hour fast from food and water the first Sunday of each month.

SECTION 2

SLEEP

We take better care of our smartphones than we do of ourselves - the phones are always recharged!

ARIANNA HUFFINGTON

A GOOD NIGHT'S SLEEP

WHEN'S THE LAST TIME you were consistently sleeping for seven to nine hours a night? Ten years ago? Twenty?

A U.S. Centers for Disease Control and Prevention report suggests that 35% of Americans are not hitting the golden number of sleep hours needed to maintain good health.[1]

A good night's sleep is usually one of the first sacrifices on the altar of success. But skipping sleep to be more productive is really just counterproductive. The evidence is straightforward... sleep deprivation leads to burnout. And ain't nobody got time for that.

After fighting her own burnout battle, Arianna Huffington, president of the Huffington Post Media Group, is leading a campaign to increase awareness and take down a corporate culture that glorifies sleep deprivation. She said:

Sleep, or how little of it we need, has become a symbol of our prowess [but,] there's practically no element of our lives that's not improved by getting adequate sleep. And there is no element of life that's not diminished by a lack of sleep.[2]

Arianna launched a company called Thrive Global with the goal to "turn sleeping well into the corporate world's most celebrated productivity tool."[3]

Sleep deprivation is not only dangerous, it's costly. In the U.S alone, researchers estimate that sleep deprivation costs us $411 billion each year due to accidents and lost productivity.[4]

As fundamental as it is, sleep is often one of the most messed with and messed up aspects of our health.

Too Little, Too Late
Sleep is the largest slice in our 24-hour pie chart and the one that we have the most control over. Does it really make a difference to shave off a couple hours of shut eye?

Well... yes. In fact, research published in the journal, *Sleep*, shows us that missing even one hour of sleep a night can have a vast impact on your health and immune system.[5] This explains why you're more likely to become sick when you're not getting enough sleep.

Scientists describe burning the candle at both ends as incurring sleep debt.[6] No executive can expect to be in the red for very long and keep the corner office. Sleep is just as unforgiving. You can't expect to keep racking up sleep debt AND maintain your health.

Most sleep doctors and scientists say that seven hours a night is the minimum recommendation and you really should be getting more.

The American Academy of Sleep Medicine (AASM) and Sleep Research Society (SRS) recommended the following:

▶ Sleeping less than 7 hours per night on a regular basis is associated with adverse health outcomes, including weight gain and obesity, diabetes, hypertension, heart disease and stroke, depression, and increased risk of death. Sleeping less than 7 hours per night is also associated with impaired immune function, increased pain, impaired performance, increased errors, and greater risk of accidents.

▶ Sleeping more than 9 hours per night on a regular basis may be appropriate for young adults, individuals recovering from sleep debt, and individuals with illnesses. For others, it is uncertain whether sleeping more than 9 hours per night is associated with health risk.[7]

If that sounds outlandish to you—maybe you've been getting by on 4 to 5 hours—you need to consider this as an investment. Luckily, this investment isn't just about long-term benefit. Immediate and short-term benefits include:

▶ Greater concentration and better overall brain function
▶ Weight loss
▶ Stronger immune system
▶ Brain and body detox

You'll also decrease your risk for some pretty major issues such as vision loss, impaired driving, diabetes, cancer, heart disease, mood disorders, Alzheimer's, migraines and hormone imbalances. A single night of sleep deprivation increases hunger hormones, which can lead to weight gain and obesity.[8]

Most of our discussions with high-performing individuals are centered around lack of sleep, however, it should be noted that too much sleep can also be a problem. Research indicates that sleeping too long may increase your risk of heart disease.[9]

In summary, sleep is a big deal. You knew that already. What you may not have known is how to do it well.

The following five chapters will introduce some proven methods and good ideas to help you obtain a better night's sleep, both in quantity and quality. We are going to talk about circadian rhythms, sleep routine, bedroom detox, and how nutrition and genetics affect your sleep.

SLEEP CULTURE

#1: Circadian Reset

Align your sleep and wake cycles to work with nature instead of against it.

#2: Sleep Routines

Routines can determine the quality of your nights and your days.

#3: Detox Your Bedroom

Bedtime and your bedroom should feel different and special.

#4: Food + Sleep

The things that we eat and drink are integral to promoting sustainable sleep and energy levels.

#5: Know Your Weaknesses

Evaluate to find any weaknesses and create a personalized plan to compensate.

HABIT #1

CIRCADIAN RESET

Align your sleep and wake cycles to work with nature instead of against it.

CIRCADIAN RESET

You've heard of circadian rhythm before. It's a real thing. And a really big thing if you're into optimizing performance.

Think about it this way: we all had that one roommate in college who played their music way too loud. Trying to chill to your own music while it's being overpowered with Metallica's Greatest Hits just doesn't really work out. It's almost impossible to feel calm, focused, and motivated. Instead you are left feeling anxious, uninspired, and confused.

Does that sound familiar? If you want to feel less anxious and confused and more inspired, focused, and motivated, perhaps you have two different rhythms going and you need to figure out which one you're going to listen to. We vote for muting the "self-made" rhythm and going for the God-given one. We all know He's smarter anyway, why fight it?

So, what is this God-given, circadian rhythm we speak of? Circadian rhythm is a 24-hour cycle observed in the physiological processes of all living things, from human life down to fungus and bacteria (including the fungus and bacteria that live inside our digestive systems). Basically, it's the boss with the watch that regulates your internal body clock, body temperature, hormones, hunger, digestion and metabolism, heart function, cell regeneration, and fatigue.[10]

Everything in nature is cyclical and our circadian rhythms are our daily cycles. When our daily cycles are off, it creates a domino effect and throws off our monthly and yearly cycles as well. Restoring homeostasis in your day rebalances your month and year. Because who needs an off year?

9 SIGNS YOU'RE OFF YOUR CIRCADIAN RHYTHM

Also known in the medical world as Circadian Rhythm Sleep Disorder, problems with your sleep-wake cycle can contribute to a host of issues that affect productivity:

1. Difficulty getting to sleep

2. Difficulty staying asleep

3. Not feeling well-rested even when you do sleep

4. Daytime sleepiness

5. Difficulty concentrating

6. Decreased cognitive skills

7. Poor coordination

8. Headaches

9. Gastrointestinal distress (including bloating, cramping, gas, irregular bowel movements)

In addition to the central clock in our brain, researchers have discovered that we have clocks controlling other parts of our bodies as well.[11] In fact, a 2017 Nobel Prize was awarded to these researchers for discovering a gene that controls circadian behavior.

When awarding them the prize, the secretary of the Nobel Assembly stated: "Studies have also indicated that chronic misalignment between our lifestyles and the clock is associated with increased risk for various diseases."[12]

CNN added that "The [Nobel] committee explained how an imbalance between lifestyle and rhythm could lead to increased risk for a number of diseases including metabolic diseases, such as diabetes and cancer, and neurodegenerative diseases, such as Alzheimer's disease."[13]

The early hours of sleep are critical, and missing that window causes your rebuilding functions to take a rain check. Why is the timing important? Sleep scientists have demonstrated that we typically sleep in 90-minute cycles that are made up of REM (Rapid Eye Movement) and non-REM phases.[14] The first half of the night is so essential because that is when we spend more time in stage 3 non-REM sleep—a deeper sleep.[15,16]

Depriving ourselves of that deep sleep can negatively affect several areas of our health, including how memories are stored. What happens if you miss that window for days… or weeks? You can see how the quality of your sleep can make or break your mental and physical performance.

Trying to reconnect with your circadian rhythms is basically just getting your body back in tune with nature. Adjust your sleep schedule with the seasons, going to sleep earlier when it gets dark earlier. If you spend enough time outside, you'll notice that you will naturally gravitate towards that schedule. If you have ever been camping, you know that it's pretty difficult to "sleep in" when you're sleeping in a tent!

When we spend our whole lives indoors under bright lights, our internal clocks become confused. Spending time outside in the morning (especially morning[17]), mid-day and evening light will help your body to rediscover its circadian rhythms.

Early to Bed, Early to Rise

You've heard Ben Franklin's famous common-sense proverb that has been repeated by mother's everywhere: "Early to bed and early to rise, makes a man healthy, wealthy, and wise".

Arguably two of the most productive figures in ancient and modern history, Aristotle and Benjamin Franklin were on the same wavelength.

Aristotle is credited with saying, "It is well to be up before daybreak, for such habits contribute to health, wealth, and wisdom."

Who are we to disagree with the collective wisdom of a pre-eminent philosopher, one of the greatest scientific and political minds in American history, and your mother?

If you require more credible credentials backing this advice, look to scripture that teaches "cease to sleep longer than is needful; retire to thy bed early, that ye may not be weary; arise early, that your bodies and minds may be invigorated."[18]

JET LAG:
6 TIPS FOR RESETTING CIRCADIAN RHYTHM WHEN TRAVELING.

Jet lag is a common plague among business leaders. According to Dr. Charles A. Czeisler, director of the Division of Sleep Medicine at Harvard Medical School, jet lag is due to a misalignment between the external environment and the internal clock in the brain that drives our daily performance, alertness, and ability to sleep.[19]

How to minimize the effects of jet lag:

1. Stay hydrated. Drink a lot of water. Avoid soda, caffeine, and alcohol, as they promote dehydration.

2. Fast before and during travel.[20]

3. Get out in the sun as soon as possible after landing.

4. Utilize the theory of grounding/earthing. Spend time connecting with the earth by walking barefoot on the beach or in the park. The slight negative charge in the earth helps neutralize the buildup of positive (i.e. energy sapping) charge in your body.

5. Get on the new schedule right when you start travelling. You may feel like a walking zombie initially but go to bed and wake up on local time.

6. Take melatonin at target destination bedtime. Studies show that melatonin is "remarkably effective in preventing or reducing jet-lag"[21]

27 YEARS OLD, Jake been hospitalized twice in the last two months for psychosis. His symptoms at the time of hospitalization included paranoia, visual and auditory hallucinations, and extreme confusion.

After some digging, I discovered that Jake and his college roommate were working on a new business venture that was taking up all of his time and focus outside of school. Jake acknowledged that his eating and sleeping habits had not been ideal.

In fact, he eventually admitted that prior to the first hospitalization, he hadn't slept for three days straight. He then drove a few hours south to a large city and was found wandering the streets in the middle of the night, trying to "drum up interest in [his] new business plans."

Jake suffered similar, though less extreme, sleep deprivation leading up to his second hospitalization. There were also a number of other stressors in his life. The second hospital stay added more diagnoses (bipolar disorder, anxiety, schizophrenia, and schizoaffective disorder), and additional potent medications. According to Jake's parents, the medications were sedating him and completely blunting his personality.

Their hope was to figure out what was really going on and reduce the prescription medicines that were robbing him of his personality and motivation. Of course, coming off that class of medications isn't something that should ever be done quickly or without close medical supervision.

After consulting together, we decided to make Jake's sleep our primary focus, while also working on his nutrition and stress management strategies. To help Jake improve his sleep, we started supplementing with magnesium and discussed some basic tips to reset his circadian rhythm. These tips include maintaining a consistent sleep schedule, avoiding exposure to blue light at least one hour before bedtime, and avoiding naps during the day.

The changes were slow, but at a follow-up visit four weeks later, Jake reported that his sleep had improved dramatically and that he had a lot more energy during the day.

He was still taking the hefty prescription medications, including antipsychotic and anti-anxiety drugs, so his brain was still fuzzy and he was still feeling somewhat sedated during the day, but noticing improvements. As his energy returned, he felt ready to exercise again, boosting his sleep quality even more.

Although we hit a few bumps in the road—which aren't unusual when dealing with powerful prescriptions—we were able to wean Jake off all his medications. He is managing incredibly well on an easily sustainable nutritional plan, regular exercise, and a few botanical supplements.

Jake's story illustrates the power and necessity of sleep in our lives. His life took a very dramatic downturn for several months because he neglected this critical need for too long. Jake and his parents were told by multiple psychiatrists that he would likely require long-term antipsychotic medications.

By adjusting his lifestyle, Jake has been able to avoid side effects and dependence on mind-altering medications and return to functioning as a normal college student. (Although let's be honest, his healthy sleep and nutrition habits are now well above those of his peers.)

Align your sleep and wake cycles to work with nature instead of against it.

NEW HABIT FORMATION

Write down the habit you would like to incorporate, including when you will do it. Whenever possible, pair the desired habit with an existing habit. For situational habits designate an if...then clause.

EXAMPLES

- We will get 8 hours of sleep each night by going to bed by 10 pm and waking up by 6 am.

- We will turn down the lights in the evening to help our bodies recognize that it's time to prepare for sleep.

HABIT #2

SLEEP ROUTINES

Those brief windows of time right before going to sleep and right after waking up determine the quality of your night and the quality of your day. Make them count!

SLEEP ROUTINES

A big part of tuning into your circadian rhythms is developing a sleep routine. You may already do this for your kids with nightly rituals like reading a book, saying prayers, telling bedtime stories, and tucking them in.

Treat yourself to a power-down hour each night before bed as well! Incorporate experiences and actions that will help you relax and detox your mind. It can include things such as reading, yoga, taking a walk, or a calming bath.

We love to spend 30 minutes in the sauna in the evening, reading, talking, or meditating. Spending your last waking hour together, whether side-by-side or interacting (and yes, you can take that however you want), helps you let go of stress and anxiety that builds up during the day.

Before you go to sleep, plan to review your day by writing in a journal—noting your wins of the day and ending your evening with gratitude. Follow that up with some time spent in prayer and meditation. Share your wins and your gratitude with God.

Waking Routine
Just like how you choose to wind down affects your sleep quality, how you choose to wake up affects the quality of the rest of your day.

If your wake-up routine consists of hitting the snooze button, that's a sure sign that you need more sleep—but on the front end, not the back end!

Many people find that they are most productive in the early hours of the day. Creating a morning routine that provides immediate benefits (i.e. makes you feel good afterwards) can help motivate you to get out of bed.

Minimize Barriers

If the snooze button is a barrier to your morning success, get an alarm clock without the option.

Lay out your yoga mat and clothes the night before to eliminate any additional steps that might keep you from getting to "downward dog."

If you plan to study right when you wake up, store your scriptures on your desk in your bedroom.

And most of all, keep yourself from getting sucked into email, social media, or news right when you wake up. Those distractions will make you feel groggy and interrupt your positivity and productivity.

Consistency is Key

It's best to go to bed and wake up at the same time each day. A set bedtime can be harder when you have teenagers, and obviously there will always be adjustments to the rule, but if you can follow it *most* of the time, then you'll have better results *most* of the time.

A 2016 study showed that fluctuating sleep times coincided with increased emotional and behavioral problems.[22] Another study done by researchers at Duke, just last year, cites issues such as high blood pressure, obesity, and increased diabetes risk in adult participants with irregular sleep/wake schedules.[23]

Even if your lifestyle requires a fluctuating bedtime, you can still control when you start your day. Starting off your morning with consistency is an important way to stay aligned with your circadian rhythms.

Getting up before the sun should be your rule of thumb. For many, any time spent in bed after the sun comes up doesn't make them feel more well-rested, no matter what time they went to bed.

Chances are, if you snooze past sunrise, you'll wake up as one of the seven dwarfs of sleeping in: groggy, foggy, moody, achy, hungry, grumpy and—ironically—still sleepy.

HABIT #2: SLEEP ROUTINES

Routines can determine the quality of your nights and your days.

NEW HABIT FORMATION

Write down the habit you would like to incorporate, including when you will do it. Whenever possible, pair the desired habit with an existing habit. For situational habits designate an if...then clause.

EXAMPLES

- We will spend 30 minutes meditating every night before bed.

- As soon as the alarm goes off in the morning, we will turn on the lamp, say our prayers, and spend 10 minutes reading the scriptures.

_____

_____

_____

_____

_____

_____

_____

_____

_____

_____

_____

_____

_____

HABIT #3

DETOX YOUR BEDROOM

Bedtime and your bedroom should feel different and special. Keep the rest of the world out of it.

DETOX YOUR BEDROOM

If you identify with the 95% of Americans that report using an electronic device within an hour of hitting the sack, that might be the best place to start in addressing your sleep issues.[24]

Looking at a screen before bedtime messes with your brain and sabotages your sleep. Even small amounts of blue light (phone, tablet, computer, TV) can drastically decrease your body's ability to produce melatonin and throw off your circadian rhythm.[25,26,27]

In a study of 10,000 teens, the more screen time they had during the day, the harder it was for them to fall asleep. Participants who used devices over five hours a day were over three times more likely to sleep for less than five hours at night and almost 50% more likely to take an hour to fall asleep.[28]

Another study of 653 adult participants concluded:

> Longer average screen-time was associated with shorter sleep duration and worse sleep-efficiency. Longer average screen-times during bedtime and the sleeping period were associated with poor sleep quality, decreased sleep efficiency, and longer sleep onset latency.[29]

If you spend your last waking minutes flipping through your phone or using Netflix as your bedtime routine, you may be missing out on the deep restorative sleep that your brain and body need to give you optimal performance the next day. Something as simple as changing your evening habits could change your life.

Minimize EMF

While it's probably not viable (for most people) to sleep in a faraday cage or shut off power to your bedroom each night, any way that you can minimize electromagnetic field (EMF) exposure is likely to help.

1. Turn off your Wi-Fi router at night.

2. Use an alarm clock (preferably battery powered) instead of your phone and keep your phone in another room.

3. Minimize electronics in your room. Ditch the TV in the bedroom, and for so many more reasons than just limiting EMF's!

4. Avoid electric blankets or heating pads.

5. Move your bed away from the wall. Wiring in walls can emit a magnetic field.

6. Replace fluorescent light bulbs in your bedroom with full spectrum incandescent lights. Avoid LED lights in the evening.[30,31]

Lights Out

Sunset signals your brain that it's time to prepare for bed. If you interrupt that natural signaling with bright lights, particularly white and blue lights that simulate daylight, it makes it harder to fall asleep. It's wise to keep lighting low and in the warm tones (yellow, orange, and red wavelengths that you'd find in a campfire) in the evening.

If you ever wake up during the night, you'll want to make sure you only turn on very dim, warm lights, because bright lights and blue lights suppress melatonin production.[32]

Once it's time for lights out, make sure it is completely dark. If you really need a clock visible, use one with red light instead of blue or white. The darker your room, the more complete the message to your brain that it is time to sleep. Skip the nightlight and bring in blackout curtains if needed.

A recent study showed that your sleep environment can have a major impact your weight. Artificial light exposure (including from a TV or computer) while sleeping is linked to significantly higher risk of obesity in women.[33]

Cool It

The optimal sleeping temperature is shown to be around 65-67 degrees. Pull out your tech savvy and schedule your thermostat to drop in temperature during the night and heat back up just before waking to make it easier to get out of bed in the morning.

Your brain's thermostat lowers at night as it prepares your body for sleep. Your core body temperature stays low until just before waking. Any disruption to this optimal sleep temperature negatively affects your sleep. According to researchers, "poor sleep is associated with elevated core body temperature."[34]

It's also important to make sure your bedroom isn't too cold, causing muscle contraction and sabotaging your ability to relax. Supporting your body's preferred sleeping temperature by making sure your home isn't too hot or too cold will increase REM and slow wave sleep and keep you from waking up at night.[35]

Fresh Is Best

A little air circulation can help keep your body temperature regulated. Fresh air at night can help keep an optimal balance of CO_2 and help you sleep deeper, more efficiently, and with less interruption.

A 2015 study reported an increased ability to concentrate, less sleepiness, and higher performance on a logical thinking test when participants opened their windows at night to promote outdoor air supply and lower CO_2 levels.[36]

The study authors estimated that exposure to poor air quality is up to sixteen times higher in the bedroom and determined that this can have a marked impact on sleep quality.

For some, sleeping with the window open might expose them sleep disruptors like a blaring siren or an overzealous rooster. White noise can help mask environmental noises and allow you to sleep better. We keep a white noise machine in an adjacent bathroom to minimize electronics near our sleeping area.[37]

Air pollution or climate might be a reason for some people to keep their windows closed. If you live in a place where you can't crack the window at night, a fan can help you at least get some air flow and a houseplant or two can improve the air quality.[38]

4 SENSES OF SLEEP

1. TACTILE: WEIGHTED BLANKETS AND COOLING SHEETS

Weighted blankets have been shown to induce a calmer night's sleep in a Swedish study involving individuals suffering from moderate insomnia.[39] Participants reported higher-quality sleep, including less movement and sleeping more comfortably and securely. Weighted blankets have become more widely available in the last few years through retailers like Amazon and Target. The recommendation is to choose a blanket that is around 10% of your body weight.

Temperature-regulating sheets that keep your body cool instead of holding in heat may help you sleep deeper. Look for textiles that absorb moisture, and that are lightweight and breathable, like organic cotton, silk, bamboo, microfiber, percale, or sateen.

2. OLFACTORY: ESSENTIAL OILS

Essential oils are one of our favorite ways to help our minds and bodies relax. The sleep-promoting benefits of essential oils have been well documented.[40,41] Essential oils have also shown to help with relieving stress and anxiety symptoms, which are often a primary factor in delaying sleep.[42,43,44]

Some of the most recommended oils for aiding in relaxation and sleep are lavender, roman chamomile, vanilla, vetiver, ylang ylang, bergamot, rose, geranium, jasmine, marjoram, cedarwood, frankincense, mandarin, and sandalwood.

Some oils can affect different people in different ways, so pay attention to how you feel and what works for you. You want to make sure that you are getting high quality oils and that you are trained on how to use essential oils safely. Essential oils are highly concentrated and should be diluted before being applied to skin.

We love using diluted oils for massage, adding a few drops to bathwater, using a diffuser in our bedroom, or mixing up a spray bottle to mist over bed linens.

One study provided personal essential oil inhaler devices called aromasticks to cancer patients. 92% reported that the using the aromastick improved their sleep and that they would continue to use it to help them sleep.[45]

3. VISUAL: HIMALAYAN SALT LAMP

A fad in the world of the health-conscious, Himalayan Salt Lamps are claimed (but not yet well studied and proven) to help mitigate indoor air pollution and neutralize electromagnetic radiation. Either way, the warm glow of a salt lamp will give you light when you need it, without shutting down your melatonin production like a white or blue light will. If you're not into salt lamps, use another soft, warm light on your bedside table.

4. AUDITORY: MUSIC

Listening to relaxing classical music in the evening can help improve your sleep quality.[46] Music that incorporates binaural beats is an "effective therapeutic tool" to increase relaxation, reduce stress, and improve sleep.[47,48,49]

In fact, in one small-scale study conducted by former president of the American Board of Anti-Aging Medicine, Dr. Vincent Giampapa, M.D., 73% of the participants had an average of 97% melatonin increase after listening to binaural beats.[50]

JEN AND STEVE are an active young couple in their 30's, both busy in their careers. One of the issues that they wanted to address when first coming to me was increased fatigue. They had problems getting to sleep and feeling rested when they woke in the morning.

Like many of us, they felt that they needed time in the evenings to relax and escape the reality of their hectic lives through Netflix binges and social media.

It took me a couple of months to convince both of them that they needed to make some fundamental changes to their nightly routine. Jen was ready to make adjustments sooner than Steve was, but going at it alone didn't work, because Steve was either working on his computer in bed or making her feel guilty about not spending time watching shows with him.

Once they were both ready to commit, we agreed to start with the two biggest steps:

1. Go to bed early and wake up early.

2. Avoid all electronics in the evening and instead do some light reading or take a walk outside together.

Within one week of implementing these changes, including consistently getting to bed by 10 pm and waking up by 5:30 or 6 am, Jen and Steve immediately noted improved sleep quality and more energy during the day. Previously, they would lay in bed for half an hour to two hours trying to fall asleep. Then they would wake up to their alarm in the morning feeling as thought they'd barely slept. Now they were both falling asleep easily and getting up rejuvenated and ready to face the day.

Jen and Steve were thrilled with this quick win. For some people it takes up to two weeks of consistent sleep schedules to reset circadian rhythms, but there are other things that you can do to speed up the reset like exercise,[51,52,53] nature time,[54] grounding,[55] and intermittent fasting, as we discussed in the nutrition section.

Bedtime and your bedroom should feel different and special.

NEW HABIT FORMATION

Write down the habit you would like to incorporate, including when you will do it. Whenever possible, pair the desired habit with an existing habit. For situational habits designate an if...then clause.

EXAMPLES

- We'll put our phones in the bathroom or another room to charge at 9 pm and leave them there until morning.

- IF we're tempted to turn on a show at night, THEN we'll go for a walk or read a book instead.

HABIT #4

F O O D   +   S L E E P

The things that
we eat and drink
are integral
to promoting
sustainable sleep
and energy levels.

FOOD + SLEEP

The things that we eat and drink impact our ability to sleep. Stimulants and sedatives are the obvious ones, but it's more than that. We're talking about the types and quality of food, the timing of when we eat, and our overall gut health.

Your gastrointestinal tract has a direct highway to your brain through the gut-brain axis.[56] In fact, the GI tract has so much control over your body that it's often called the "second brain." When you understand this, it makes sense that nutrition, gut health, and sleep are so interrelated. Both the gut and the brain produce sleep-related neurotransmitters: dopamine, serotonin, melatonin, and GABA.

Dr. Brannick Riggs, MD wrote:

> ...gut microbes shape the architecture of sleep and stress reactivity of the hypothalamic-pituitary adrenal axis. This means that the type of bacteria we have in our gastrointestinal tract changes how well we sleep, how we react to stress, and how healthy our hormonal system is. They influence memory, mood, and cognition, and are clinically and therapeutically relevant to a range of disorders. It is important for us to eat the right kinds of foods to support a healthy gut microbiome.

Gut health and sleep affect each other in such a cyclical way that making improvements to one will often improve the other.[57]

Research shows that sleep deprivation changes the gut microbiome.[58]

There are also studies showing that better sleep quality is associated with higher proportions of specific gut bacteria.[59]

A Japanese study compared two groups of students preparing to take an exam. One group was given a probiotic drink each day, while the other was given a placebo. The placebo group experienced trouble sleeping as the day of the test grew nearer.

The group given the probiotic was under the same amount of stress (same test date) but experienced far less difficulty sleeping. They were falling asleep faster, maintaining deeper sleep, and waking up more rested than the placebo group.[60]

As we eat foods that support and add diversity to our microbiome, we improve our sleep quality. As we improve our sleep, we strengthen our gut health. When we are working to optimize our nutrition and sleep hygiene (how clean/toxin-free our sleep environment is), it eliminates the desire or need for chemical stimulants and sedatives and we can avoid the associated negative consequences.

GREG WAS A VERY busy husband and father of 6 kids when he decided to go back to school to make a major career change. Initially, things were going well, but he got a little behind and the stress began to affect him more than it ever had before. He started having panic attacks and had to take a couple of semesters off before going back for his last year.

By the time Greg came to me, he was a year and a half into what was quickly becoming an overwhelmingly busy career. As we spoke, he admitted that his sleep was one of the first things he sacrificed when he was busy with school and his sleep patterns had never recovered.

Greg also shared that his eating habits were not optimal. He would grab fast food during a quick lunch and then be starving by the time he got home in the evening. He usually ended up eating large high-carb meals—mostly processed food—late at night, while trying to finish up his charts for the day.

There were a lot of aspects of Greg's lifestyle that we could focus on to help improve his sleep and health, but we opted to start simple and focused on his nutrition. I prescribed the following:

1. Plan a large breakfast in the morning with plenty of good protein, vegetables, and high-quality fats.

2. At the beginning of each week, plan meals to take for lunch that also have adequate amounts of healthy and satiating proteins, fats, and vegetables.

3. Shift lunch back two hours, to 2 pm.

4. For two days a week, don't eat any food after the 2 pm meal and instead focus on getting adequate hydration.

5. On days when still eating in the evening, make it a very light meal—a small salad, soup, or protein smoothie.

Every week or two we added one more day where Greg skipped his evening meal until he was rarely eating in the evening at all, except on special occasions (usually on weekends). Greg initially required some protein-rich snacks between morning and mid-day meals, but as his body adjusted, it became easier and easier for him.

Not only did Greg lose weight, which was one of his primary goals, but he was shocked to find that by not eating at night, his gut no longer felt heavy and he found it easier for his mind to relax and to fall asleep quickly. As a result, his energy levels improved, as did his performance at work and his ability to optimize and enjoy time with his family (which now includes seven children!).

When to Eat, When to Sleep

Resetting your eating cycles can help reset your circadian rhythm. Breakfast literally means "breaking your fast". You can reset your eating cycles and reconnect with your circadian rhythm by fasting for 16 hours before waking up and having your breakfast. That means not eating after 3 pm if you want to wake up and eat breakfast at 7 am.

In 2009, Dr. Clifford Saper and colleagues at Harvard-affiliated Beth Israel Deaconess Medical Center identified a second "master clock" in mice that can regulate circadian rhythms when food is scarce.[61] In essence, the body's circadian rhythms are suspended to conserve energy.

It's been theorized that humans may have a similar mechanism and that a brief fast may trigger a quick reset of circadian rhythms. Dr. Saper has suggested a 12-to-16-hour fast the day before and during travel.

When we decided to shift our eating window to earlier in the day, we both noticed improvements in our sleep. Amy used to wake up during the night with stomach pains several times a week, but that went away as soon as we stopped eating late.

Eating too close to bedtime puts your body into a catabolic state— breaking down sugars and muscle tissue into usable energy—instead of an anabolic state—rebuilding tissue and healing organs.

While protein is important for all the rebuilding work that happens during the night, it's harder for your body to digest protein at night. Getting your protein early in the day and keeping evening meals light will help you sleep (and rebuild) better.

Do you ever wake up hungry during the night? Eating sugars or carbs right before bedtime is the likely culprit. Your blood sugar drops a few hours after sugar consumption, and that can wake you up and make it hard to fall back asleep.

One exception to this is having a little raw honey in the evening. Raw honey can help fuel your liver and brain during the night. We often have some warm herbal tea in the evening with a teaspoon of honey, especially in the winter. Also, adding a couple tablespoons of MCT oil or coconut oil can help keep nighttime cravings away.

Mixed Messages

It's incredibly confusing to your brain when it knows it's time to gear down and prepare for sleep, but you just boosted it into overdrive with a shot of caffeine.

Give your brain a break and avoid all stimulants for at least 6 hours before bed.[62] But really, just avoid them in general if you're into optimizing your sleep and your life (i.e. if you are reading this book).

And what about alcohol? Some will tell you that it calms them down, but science says otherwise. We don't drink as a religious and personal choice (family history with alcoholism is a really good motivator), but we also advise patients to minimize their alcohol consumption as an informed, science-based choice.

Alcohol before bedtime leads to more disrupted sleep in the second half of the night and less REM sleep overall, which means you feel less rested when you wake up.[63] Also, if you are already sleep deprived and add alcohol into the mix, it exacerbates sleepiness and impairs performance the next day.[64,65]

The things that we eat and drink are integral to promoting sustainable sleep and energy levels.

NEW HABIT FORMATION
Write down the habit you would like to incorporate, including when you will do it. Whenever possible, pair the desired habit with an existing habit. For situational habits designate an if...then clause.

EXAMPLES

- We'll cut out all stimulants and sedatives and go to bed and wake up naturally.

- IF we're craving caffeine, THEN we'll drink lemon water or water kefir instead.

HABIT #5

ADDRESS YOUR WEAKNESSES

Evaluate to find any weaknesses and create a personalized plan to compensate.

ADDRESS YOUR WEAKNESSES

Nutrient and Mineral Deficiencies

Addressing nutrient and mineral deficiencies is a quick and easy way to boost your sleep. Vitamin C, vitamin D, and vitamin B12 can all impact sleep quality, as well as magnesium, potassium, and calcium. In our experience, we find magnesium, vitamin D, and vitamin B12 to be the most common deficiencies related to sleep.

One of the first things we do for our patients is run advanced lab panels to test for key nutrient deficiencies. Research indicates that nutritional deficiencies can affect performance even at levels that fit within normal reference ranges for most labs, so it is important to make sure that your doctor is trained in advanced lab interpretation.

Hormone Imbalances

We frequently run hormone tests for patients to help us evaluate if melatonin, cortisol, progesterone, estrogen, and DHEA imbalances may be affecting sleep. When appropriate, we may recommend supplementing with melatonin, 5-HTP, hormone precursors, or bio-identical hormone replacement.

Herbal Sleep Aids

We are often asked about herbal sleep aids and there are several that we recommend based on patient needs. Many natural options, including passionflower, kava tea, valerian, and roman chamomile have been used for centuries to help improve sleep problems.

Many of our patients report that CBD oil, though controversial, improves their relaxation and sleep. Glutathione and GABA precursors such as L-theanine and phenibut are additional options that we often recommend as part of a personalized nutrition and supplement plan.

As with any medication or supplement, there are possible side effects and interactions, so we recommend consulting with a doctor who has training in both natural supplements and prescription medications.

Discussing possible sleep supplements and the research behind them could take up several chapters by itself. Please visit our website for more detailed and up-to-date information.

Essential Oils

Essential oils and essential oil supplements may be helpful in calming your mind and body before bed. We like to use a blend of lavender, roman chamomile, marjoram, ylang ylang, and Hawaiian sandalwood. Wild orange and vetiver are also favorites for promoting a good night's sleep.

Lavender is the most researched essential oil, with studies showing improvement in multiple markers of sleep quality in a variety of different populations, including postpartum women[66] and younger men and women.[67]

Rose is another oil that many find helpful for enhancing sleep, with users reporting less waking during the night and other sleep benefits.

Genetics + Sleep

Genetics play a big role in sleep. In fact, researchers say that your DNA determines anywhere from 31-55% of your sleep duration.[68] Behavior and environment account for the rest—lifestyle factors addressed in the previous four habits.

If you are still experiencing sleep issues after trying the other things that we have talked about in this section, we recommend doing a genetic test like 23andme to assess for specific genetic variations which might be contributing.

CRY1

The CRY1 gene mutation is associated with a delayed melatonin release. Most individuals have circadian rhythms that set a rise in melatonin around 9-10pm. People with the CRY1 gene variant have an altered circadian cycle and don't release melatonin until later.

Results from one large genetic database show estimates that this gene mutation could affect up to one in 75 people of European (non-Finnish) descent.[69]

Focusing on circadian rhythms is critical for individuals with this variant. Strong light exposure during the day is one suggested method for realigning circadian rhythms.[70]

We often consider supplementing with L-tryptophan—a precursor for melatonin that can increase melatonin production. Cycling low-dose melatonin supplementation (a week or two on and then a week off) can also be beneficial.

FABP7

A couple of years ago, researchers at Washington State University discovered how a gene called FABP7 affects quality of sleep in animals and humans.[71] They found that, in mice, the expression of the FABP7 gene changes over the course of the day. In addition, his team found that mice with a disabled FABP7 gene had much more disrupted sleep than mice with standard FABP7 function.

This discovery raised the question of how humans might be affected by mutations in the FABP7 gene, so the team turned to a sleep study of 300 Japanese men that included analysis of their DNA. Twenty-nine men had a special variant of the FABP7 gene—one that was correlated with their sleep patterns. Those with the variant slept more fitfully and woke up more often than people with the "normal" non-variant gene.

One of our standard recommendations for affected individuals is to get to bed earlier to ensure adequate sleep.

KNOW THYSELF
Genetic testing can provide a map showing you how to avoid your specific potential health issues.

If you are aware of your genetic weaknesses, you can control lifestyle factors and take advantage of the science of epigenetics to turn on and off specific gene expression.

Look for a physician trained in genetics and epigenetic interventions that can help you read and interpret your genetic testing and make personalized recommendations according to your unique needs.

Genetic testing has become much more accessible in the last 10 years, allowing us to provide precision medicine as standard care. We are able to streamline medications, formulate diet and supplement recommendations, and provide exercise plans and sleep recommendations—all based on your DNA.

SHORTLY AFTER going through menopause, Kathy began to have difficulty falling asleep and would wake up several times throughout the night. She spent several months trying different ove the counter and prescription sleep aids, but they made no difference.

By the time Kathy came to see me, she was getting desperate. The lack of sleep was making it almost impossible to manage the stress of being a busy branch supervisor for a bank.

We started with a well-rounded approach of optimizing Kathy's nutrition, designating exercise and outdoor nature time, and working on controlling her stress levels. These all helped a little, but just temporarily and then the sleep issues returned.

We decided to do some genetic testing and look at Kathy's methylation, which shows how the body is using B vitamins.

We discovered that she had major genetic changes that meant she was only able to use about 25%-30% of the energy from B vitamins. We decided to add some methylated B vitamins to her supplement plan, along with SamE, a supplement that supports the methylation cycle.

Within two weeks, Kathy was reporting better sleep consistency.

Within two months, she was sleeping all night and felt 10 years younger.

She was able to manage the stress at work with her additional physical and mental energy and was able to find more joy and happiness in her life and marriage as a result.

Genetic testing allowed us to see exactly what Kathy needed to support her body in a specific, sustainable way and bring her back to performing at 100%.

Most cases are not this straightforward, but this is a good example of the incredible difference that genetic testing can make in insomnia and sleep health.

Evaluate to find any weaknesses and create a personalized plan to compensate.

NEW HABIT FORMATION
Write down the habit you would like to incorporate, including when you will do it. Whenever possible, pair the desired habit with an existing habit. For situational habits designate an if...then clause.

EXAMPLES

- We'll correct the magnesium deficiency that may be affecting our sleep by taking supplements each night after brushing our teeth.

- We'll get labs done at least yearly to stay on top of deficiencies or potential problems.

SECTION 3

STRESS

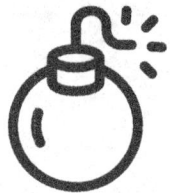

Downgrade your
fight or flight
response and
upgrade your
brain to focus
on positivity and
overcome stress.

BURNOUT CULTURE

WE LIVE IN A BURNOUT CULTURE.

Your worth is measured by how busy you are. There are a lot of rats in the race and the only way you can be at the front is to work harder, longer, and faster, right?

Maybe not. Science (and personal experience) tells us that it's not actually about working harder. It's all about working smarter. For example, most of us have noticed that when we are really stressed, we don't think as clearly.

Burnout is such a great descriptor for what so many of us experience in our jobs, both in the workplace and at home. Many shine like a match—bright for a while and then gone—sidelined by mental or physical health problems.

Overworking and overproducing isn't healthy or sustainable. But if you live responsibly—solar powering your productivity—you can shine indefinitely.

I (Scott) have vivid memories of the long, stressful, sleepless nights during residency where I was running non-stop from the ER to the ICU to Labor and Delivery. The next morning, the team of residents, medical students, and nurses rounded on all the patients with the attending physician, who was quick to highlight any flawed decisions made during the night.

Between the deadly cocktail of sleep deficit and the pressure of making life and death situations on the fly, those were some of the most stressful moments of my career.

Fortunately, I can say that all these patients survived despite our suboptimal nocturnal treatments!

Fight or Flight

Some of the most difficult cases that we see are patients who are overloaded with stress. The stress is most often related to work or relationships, and they can't seem to gain control of it.

Stress creates a constant signaling cycle in their brains that is difficult to reverse. Every day that they live in a difficult situation—experiencing conflict or worry at home or in the office—their brains are interpreting their situation as stressful and creating signals to perpetuate their fight-or-flight condition.

The stress signals go to the adrenal glands (tiny little organs sitting on top of the kidneys), which in turn release cortisol, epinephrine (adrenaline), and other stress hormones.

These hormones are important and can even be life-saving in certain situations (cue the running-away-from-a-bear analogy). However, when these fight-or-flight hormones remain chronically elevated, they wreak havoc throughout the body.

Stress Symptoms

Stress can be expressed through a host of physical symptoms. Sometimes people are so used to stress that they don't even realize that their stress hormones are constantly elevated. Stress contributes to inflammation, which is a common root cause of many health issues.

Stress-related symptoms frequently include:

- Gut issues (i.e. irritable bowel syndrome, cramping or pain, acid reflux and heartburn, nausea, irregular elimination, lack of appetite, and/or food sensitivities)

- Recurrent infections

- Back, joint and muscle pain

- Weight gain or weight loss

- Fatigue

- Insomnia

- Anxiety

- Depression

- Loss of motivation

- Brain fog, inability to concentrate, and even memory loss

- Irritability

- Hair loss

Stress Changes Your Gut

Dr. Chris Kresser recently highlighted a study showing that stress can affect your gut health as much as a poor diet can.[1] He said,

> This may explain why some patients with SIBO and other gut conditions either don't respond to treatment or do respond initially but quickly experience a return of symptoms. If stress disrupting the gut microbiome is the underlying cause of the dysfunction, then taking antimicrobials or even following special diets might help for a time, but they won't address the cause.[2]

Stress Changes Your Brain

A study published in *The Journal of the American Academy of Neurology* looked at the association between early morning cortisol levels and people's cognitive function and brain structure. The participants were younger to middle-aged adults with no reported symptoms at the onset of the study.

The people who had higher blood cortisol levels were found to have lower overall brain volumes and greater memory impairment compared to participants with average cortisol levels. This association was especially pronounced in women.[3] In other words, being stressed for a prolonged period of time can have devastating effects on our brains, potentially affecting both size and function.

Dr. Rick Hanson, a neuropsychologist, explained some possible contributing factors to stress-related brain changes at the IFM Annual International Conference in 2018. Two key concepts included negativity bias and neuroplasticity.

Negativity Bias

Negativity bias is the term scientists use to describe the innate human tendency to focus on negative experiences and stimuli. Dr. Hanson explained that this is a biologically hardwired cognitive bias engineered to help humans survive in the natural environment in which we evolved.

In earlier times, negative experiences were usually threats to human survival, so those most attentive to threats were the most likely to live another day to pass their genes down. Positive experiences—while enjoyable—didn't enhance odds of survival and therefore didn't mandate as much attention in the brain.

Dr. Hanson puts it this way: our brains are like Teflon for positive experiences and Velcro for negative ones. If this sounds like a recipe for unhappiness, well … it is, and it's one reason that depression and anxiety are epidemic in the modern world.

I know this is beginning to sound hopeless, so it's time for the good news:

We can rewire our brains for positivity and happiness!

Neuroplasticity

Neuroplasticity is the proven principle that we can change the structure and function of our brains through thoughts, emotions, and behavior. Incredible, right?

This means that we can overcome our inherent negativity bias and literally rewire our brains to pay more attention to positive experiences and less attention to negative ones.

Negativity bias leads to unhappiness, anxiety, and depression. Positivity bias results in happiness, contentedness, and zest for life.

Luckily, rewiring your brain is not as hard as it sounds. We'll show you how.

We are going to share strategies for training your brain to overcome stress and negativity bias throughout this section, and in the following section on purpose and commitment.

In this section, we will discuss how to identify your stress, how to address the root causes of stress and how to improve your body's response to stress through meditation, exercise, and spending time in nature.

KELLY AND PHIL decided to leave a busy California lifestyle and resettle in Southern Utah. Unfortunately, within a few months of arriving, Kelly began second-guessing their decision.

She was missing her friends and family. She was used to working full time, and now she didn't know how to fill her days. She couldn't tolerate the summer heat of Southern Utah. She was spending most of her time inside and starting to have symptoms of depression, anxiety, and insomnia, difficulty with memory and concentration, and extreme fatigue.

Kelly and Phil searched for activities and treatments that might help and tried a lot of things without success. By the time they came in to see us, Kelly was only sleeping a few hours a night, crying every day, and didn't want to leave the house. All she could think about was moving back home.

Phil was supportive, trying everything he could to help Kelly. He was even getting ready to re-list their new home so they could move back to California. Fortunately, Kelly and Phil had a very strong relationship, which Kelly viewed as her primary source of strength.

After discovering some deficiencies and inflammation in Kelly's labs, we developed a personalized plan of action that included a strict elimination diet, mood-boosting nutraceuticals, and more outdoor time.

Four weeks later, Kelly came back in looking and acting like a completely different person. She appeared radiant, happy, and healthy—and so did Phil. They both lost weight and seemed to have a lot more energy, but the difference was much bigger than that.

By diving into the recommended treatment plan together, they were united in their purpose and became stronger as a couple. Their nutrition improved significantly, and they enjoyed spending time together preparing and eating good food. They also spent a lot more time outside and treasured their walks together.

Kelly's mindset changed as they worked together to change their lifestyle, and this helped her to focus forward and have a more positive outlook on the things that previously brought stress.

In just four weeks of this new lifestyle, everything had changed.

In the months before, the stress of starting a new life without friends and family—along with losing the stress-relieving outdoor time she was used to—shifted Kelly's microbiome. Traumatic experiences earlier in her life combined with years of eating a less-than-ideal diet made her more susceptible to the gut issues that contribute to anxiety, depression, and insomnia. The new stress tipped her over the edge.

Kelly and Phil's relationship was the foundation for her improvement. When we were able to add in a new purpose and reason to work together and then build nutrition and lifestyle changes on top of that, results came quickly.

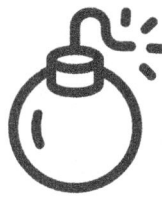

STRESS-FREE CULTURE

#1: Identify Your Stress
Analyze and record your underlying stressors.

#2: Fix What Is Fixable
Courage to change the things you can.

#3: Take Back Control
*Utilize "time-outs" to clear
and refocus your mind.*

#4: Exercise
Moving more means stressing less.

#5: Nature
Healing has its roots in nature.

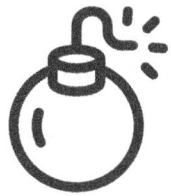

HABIT #1

IDENTIFY YOUR STRESS

Analyze and record your underlying stressors.

IDENTIFY YOUR STRESS

The first step in dealing with stress is to figure out what's causing it. This may seem obvious, but it is often overlooked or rarely allocated adequate time and effort.

Identifying the sources of your stress requires regular honest self-evaluation and introspection. As you ponder potential stressors, consider the following questions:

- Am I letting matters that are out of my control stress me out?

- Am I using my time wisely?

- Is there anything about my physical appearance that upsets me?

- Do I regularly feel guilt over something in my life?

- Do I spend time comparing what I accomplish, who I am, or what I have with others?

- Is there a mismatch in my life right now between who I want to be and who I currently see myself as?

- Am I thinking negative thoughts before I fall asleep?

- Am I moving toward or away from my ultimate goals and dreams?

- Am I living true to myself and the things I hold to be important?

- Do I feel like I'm letting down somebody who I care about?

Ask for Help

You may find it helpful to discuss these questions as a couple, and also with trusted friends, family, and others. Ask each person for help in discovering what your underlying stressors are, because sometimes others have insights about us that we haven't yet recognized or even considered.

It's important to be honest and sincere with one another, and more important (and often more difficult) to be open to hearing and considering what others have to share. A humble willingness to be vulnerable is key to discovering the root cause of your stress.

Prayer is a critical part of the process. Taking the opportunity to ask God can yield surprising answers.

Write down your own thoughts, suggestions from others, and the inspiration you receive from heaven. The list may be short—one or two items—or it may fill a whole page. It doesn't matter. You only need to work on one item at a time.

Remove Stress

Pick a starting point and challenge yourself to do a little better tomorrow than you did today. The true marker of success is that we climb. It doesn't matter how fast or slow we go—only that we are moving upward.

For some, it makes sense to attempt to tackle the biggest stressor on the list first. However, we most commonly recommend picking something from your list that you know you can address easily and then gain momentum from a quick win.

Analyze and record your underlying stressors.

NEW HABIT FORMATION

Write down the habit you would like to incorporate, including when you will do it. Whenever possible, pair the desired habit with an existing habit. For situational habits designate an if...then clause.

EXAMPLES

- When we record the week in our journals, we'll identify any new or persisting stressors in our lives that need to be addressed.

- We'll be mindful of our feelings in the moment. IF we catch ourselves feeling stressed, THEN we'll stop, identify the stressor, and categorize it to be dealt with appropriately.

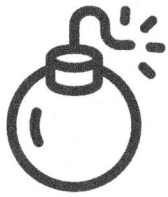

HABIT #2

FIX WHAT IS FIXABLE

"God grant me the serenity to accept the things I cannot change, courage to change the things I can, and wisdom to know the difference."

- Reinhold Niebuhr

FIX WHAT IS FIXABLE

We advocate an annual "State of the Stress" address. As you consider the influences in your life—how they align with your soul purpose and how they may be affecting your health—there might be some very difficult decisions to be made.

You may need to consider a change at work (or even a complete career change). You might decide to talk to a supervisor about shifting your responsibilities or who you work directly with. You might resolve to let a problematic employee go, hire someone to relieve some of your workload, or you and your spouse may decide to simplify your life so that one of you can work from home or stop working.

These are all major changes to make, but when you have a clear vision of what you want, it makes hard choices more doable. We've worked with courageous people who, once they realized the impact of stress in their lives, have chosen to make some drastic life changes.

One brave patient, with the encouragement of her husband, left her job at a local nursery, where she worked for 12 years, and started her own business. She had always dreamed of doing it, but never dared to try until she realized that her previous job was affecting her health and she needed a change.

Another woman was working three different jobs to take some financial pressure off her husband, but she was exhausted. She explained that her ultimate goal was to be able to focus on what she really loved, which was real estate.

We ordered some hormone testing to see how she was functioning. Once she saw that her lab results showed elevated cortisol levels and lots of inflammation, she had all the motivation she needed. She reported at our next visit that she quit her other jobs and dove into real estate full-time.

If you're not sure if your stress is work-related, pay close attention to your stress levels on days off. Think back to how you felt during and after your last vacation. If you don't remember your last vacation, that's probably a sign that you need to plan one (in the name of scientific discovery, of course!) We've had many patients who have come back after a vacation excited that their primary symptoms (headaches, brain fog, fatigue, insomnia, or anxiety) seemed to disappear while they were gone. That's invaluable insight to gain!

It is critical to recognize that you are in charge of your life.

You are in charge of your stress levels.

While there may occasionally be external circumstances that you cannot change, you have the internal power to change every situation you find yourself in, even if it is only your response or your outlook.

In situations where we can't immediately find a solution, the solution may be to seek support in learning how to shift our outlook and better handle our stress.

One of our great mentors and friends, Illens Dort, wrote about solving problems. He said:

> Problems that can be solved offer us an opportunity to exercise our mental capacity. Problems that can't be solved offer us an opportunity to exercise our faith.[4]

The Biology of Stress

We are wired to perform in stressful moments. The body's automatic reaction to a threat is instantaneous and powerful. However, if stressful moments start to run together into stress-filled days, weeks, and months, problems arise. We are engineered for brief bursts of danger, not a constant, chronic threat to our well-being.

If you are always worried about problems at work or dealing with a lot of stress at home, your body may reach the point where the stress signaling cycle (the HPA axis) begins to run awry. Chronic stress hijacks the normally beneficial acute stress response.

Your body responds to acute stress with a rapid release of hormones (cortisol and adrenaline), followed by an appropriate inhibitory signal to allow the body to recover. Chronic stress doesn't allow recovery time and, inevitably, your body will begin to feel the effects. This can affect each of us in a different way.

In addition, if your brain interprets that you're in a stressful situation, your body will reserve all energy to fight or flee from a potential threat. It's not going to waste any energy on other tasks. This is why one of the most common symptoms of stress is fatigue.

Imagine that you survive a plane crash in the middle of the ocean. You're fortunate enough to find a paddle board among the debris, but salvage only one piece of luggage. You must decide how you will use those resources to help you survive as long as possible. If you blow through the beef jerky stash in the first two days, you're likely to starve—so you have to ration it. You're also not going to be doing your usual intense paddleboard yoga or you'll burn too many precious calories.

In the same way, when your body feels it might need every ounce of energy to deal with a threat (perceived or real), it won't exhaust energy on anything that's not critical for survival.

CORTISOL AND IMMUNE FUNCTION

As cortisol rises, it blocks your immune system's protective effects, making you more susceptible to catching whatever bug is going around. You start to notice you get sick more than you used to, and never quite feel like you're completely over it. You are more prone to getting illnesses like Mono, shingles, cold sores (caused by the herpes virus), and a host of others. Inappropriately blunting the immune response even puts people at a higher risk of major diseases such as cancer,[5,6,7,8] heart attacks,[9,10,11] and strokes.[12,13]

CORTISOL & HORMONES

A hormone is a chemical messenger in our body that is produced by a gland, such as the thyroid, testicles, ovaries, adrenal glands, and even the pancreas (insulin) and the kidneys (vitamin D), and then transported through the blood to act on other areas in the body.

Abnormal levels of cortisol can limit the ability of hormones—like estrogen, progesterone, and testosterone—to work properly.[14,15]

Many patients come in with complaints of hormonal abnormalities and requesting hormone replacement therapy. Most of the time it's true—their hormones are out of whack. However, I always like to consider what is causing the hormonal roller coaster, instead of immediately jumping into the same conventional medicine approach of a pill (or cream) for every ill. We usually test hormone levels via urine or saliva to see how the adrenal glands are functioning.

Almost invariably, if the reproductive hormone levels are off, so are the cortisol and/or DHEA levels (both released by the adrenal glands). There are medications that can be taken to support the adrenals, and often they can be helpful, but we still aren't getting to the root of the issue that way.

The only sustainable way to fix adrenal and hormonal abnormalities caused by stress is to address the root cause of the stress.

Goals versus Reality Disconnect

A major source of stress for many of us is the realization that the road we are currently on is not going to lead us toward our goals. Some examples of this include the following:

- Wishing you had a different career.

- Wanting to be healthier or lose weight but recognizing that you're eating a processed food diet and living a sedentary life.

- Viewing yourself as a kind and loving person but realizing that you're not treating the people close to you (spouse, kids, friends, co-workers) the way you know you should.

- Desiring to further develop (or at least maintain) skills and talents, but never making the time to do so.

- Wishing you could be a parent who spends time developing strong relationships with your kids, but then never making time with family a priority.

- Wishing that you could increase your knowledge but never taking the time to study and learn.

If you find any of these are true for you, it's time to make a change. If there are multiple disconnects in your life, pick the one you're most ready to change and do it! You may be intimidated or even terrified. It may require some big adjustments to your life. You may not know where to start. The answer is...just start!

A phrase frequently used by a couple of our mentors that really hits home for us is: imperfect action is better than no action. We have felt frozen by the fear of not being able to produce perfection—like when we began writing this book. Procrastination doesn't lead to perfection—just more stress.

When you jump in and start trying, you'll find that momentum wins. To quote another common phrase, done is better than perfect.

Divine Discontent

While comparison and guilt are negative emotions, there is a healthy side to recognizing when we fall short. When we realize that we are not doing what we should and feel a pull to change and do better, that motivating factor is beneficial and even crucial. Religious leader Neal A. Maxwell termed this feeling "Divine Discontent."

Michelle Craig spoke on this theme, saying,

> Divine discontent comes when we compare 'what we
> are [to] what we have the power to become.' Each of
> us, if we are honest, feels a gap between where and
> who we are, and where and who we want to become.
> We yearn for greater personal capacity...These feel-
> ings are God given and create an urgency to act.[16]

Guilt and comparison drag us down and make us feel hopeless, but
divine discontent does the opposite. Recognizing the gap between
who we are and who we can be is a hopeful exercise that inspires improvement and enables the process of perfection (which is an eternal
promise—not one that is met in this brief life).

We don't need to feel stressed, trapped, or discouraged by our mortal
weaknesses. The enabling power of the atonement of Jesus Christ can
transform our efforts and make up the difference.

Divine discontent supplies the energy to step out of our comfort zone
and continue to push ourselves. This is true in every aspect of our
lives and in all of our interactions—in our careers, in our communi-
ties, and especially in our homes.

We should never expect that life will always be easy and comfortable
(that's not why we're here!), but we can expect that we have been
given the capacity to handle struggles and threats when they come.
The important thing is to recognize when we are hampering that ability by filling our lives with self-induced stress or situations that we
have the capacity to change, if we are willing.

Each time we feel stressed we need to consider if we are being weighed down by guilt and debilitating discouragement because we are not measuring up to our own unreasonable expectations. We will often have to drop something in our lives as we prioritize those activities that carry eternal significance.

Clean Up Your Life

If you want to reduce stress in your life, a great place to start is to reduce the things that are cluttering up your days, your thoughts, or your home.

ACTIVITIES

Do you have too many good things going? Is over scheduling and overcommitting a common theme in your life?

In a talk titled, "Good, Better, Best" Dallin Oaks said:

> Just because something is good is not a sufficient reason for doing it. The number of good things we can do far exceeds the time available to accomplish them. Some things are better than good, and these are the things that should command priority attention in our lives. … We have to forego some good things in order to choose others that are better or best.[17]

For some of us, busy is a badge of honor, signaling a disconnect in our lives about where our worth really comes from.

When we heap obligations upon ourselves in an effort to build up our perceived value, we end up buried in a mountain of stress—because we're not even doing these things for the right reasons.

For others, being busy is a form of what Brene Brown terms numbing. She said:

> 'Crazy-busy' is a great armor, it's a great way for numbing. What a lot of us do is that we stay so busy, and so out in front of our life, that the truth of how we're feeling and what we really need can't catch up with us.[18]

Are we compensating for a lack of purpose by filling our lives with busyness and stress?

The magnifying glass of deeper meaning allows us to view our schedules with clarity so we can judge which activities serve as distractions, shields, false pedestals, and ultimately, unnecessary stressors.

Saying yes to something always means saying no to something else. It's easier to be wise about accepting invitations or assignments when you identify what you'll be giving up.

In his book, Essentialism, leadership and business expert, Greg McKeown, makes a great case for only spending time on the things that matter most. He says,

> It's about challenging the core assumption of 'we can have it all' and 'I have to do everything' and replacing it with the pursuit of 'the right thing, in the right way, at the right time'. It's about regaining control of our own choices about where to spend our time and energies instead of giving others implicit permission to choose for us.[19]

NUMBING

Ironically, a lot of the things that people do to "de-stress" are really just forms of numbing. The unspoken motive behind these unproductive activities is to keep us from thinking and feeling.

These bad habits end up sucking up time and brain capital, robbing us of the opportunity to invest in true stress-reducing habits—and, ultimately, greater success.

Do you ever find yourself thinking about what's going to happen in the next episode of that new series you are addicted to? Or constantly checking to see how your March Madness bracket is performing? Have you ever fallen into the rabbit hole of useless YouTube videos and completely lost track of time?

You could fill a landfill with the research documenting the detrimental effects of living out your social life online and the amount of time wasted there.

What about listening to music that isn't uplifting or reading the latest celebrity gossip? Do these things add or diffuse stress in your life?

Our stress is affected by everything that we allow into our lives, so it's imperative to be selective.

Clean Up Your Home

Just thinking about cleaning your house might make you feel overwhelmed but simplifying your life and your surroundings down to essentials is a clear-cut way to reduce stress in the long run.

Working and living in a clean and calm environment promotes peace, joy, and creativity in all areas of life.

Researchers at Indiana University found that people with clean houses tend to be healthier and more active than people with messy houses.[20]

A 2010 study applied linguistic analysis software to recordings of women describing their homes. Women who used words like "cluttered" were more likely to be depressed and fatigued than women who used descriptions like "restful" and "restorative." Researchers also found that women with cluttered homes had flatter patterns of cortisol release, which is associated with several adverse health outcomes.[21]

We highly recommend Marie Kondo's book, *The Life-Changing Magic of Tidying Up*. The basic premise of the book is that you empty your home (in steps) and then only put back the things that spark joy.

How would it feel to look around your home and only see items that bring you joy?

Imagine how much that could enable creativity in your life! Clutter drags us down, filling our mind and zapping our energy. We need that energy and creativity to find the success we desire.

Waking up in a clean bedroom gives you the best possible start to your day. In fact, people who make their beds are 19% more likely to report a good night's sleep and 70% said they sleep better when their sheets are freshly cleaned.[22]

Now, there may be some of you who are so obsessed with keeping your home clean that you can't ever seem to relax. If that's true for you, then perhaps as you review the following suggestions you may be inspired to recognize that a few of your current daily routines are less critical. Sometimes it's good to tidy up your cleaning routine too!

Clean Up Your Thoughts

Is there anything weighing on your mind or keeping you up at night?

Thoughts that hijack our brains during downtime are often anxiety related. Worry about things on our long-term to-do list (the one we never seem to get to!) or current events can interrupt our sleep. Having 72-hour kits in place, essential food and supplies stored for emergencies, and adequate insurance can help free up mental space that can be used for more productive things.

What about mental energy spent rehashing bad conversations, reliving injustices, and dwelling on negativity?

Back in 2007, James E. Faust quoted Dr. Sidney Simon, sharing the following wisdom about forgiveness:

> Dr. Sidney Simon, a recognized authority on values realization, has provided an excellent definition of forgiveness as it applies to human relationships:
>
> 'Forgiveness is freeing up and putting to better use the energy once consumed by holding grudges, harboring resentments, and nursing unhealed wounds. It is rediscovering the strengths we always had and relocating our limitless capacity to understand and accept other people and ourselves' [with Suzanne Simon, Forgiveness: How to Make Peace with Your Past and Get on with Your Life (1990), 19].[23]

COMPARISON AND UNREALISTIC EXPECTATIONS

Comparison is a common cause of stress for people we meet, because it's so difficult to avoid. From the time we are young, we are entrenched in a comparison culture. When we don't feel like we measure up, we can feel stressed or depressed.

In an address in 2011, religious leader Dieter Uchtdorf wisely counseled,

> We spend so much time and energy comparing ourselves to others—usually comparing our weaknesses to their strengths. This drives us to create expectations for ourselves that are impossible to meet. As a result, we never celebrate our good efforts because they seem to be less than what someone else does...Many of you are endlessly compassionate and patient with the weaknesses of others. Please remember also to be compassionate and patient with yourself.[24]

This is especially true in today's social media world, where we have unlimited access to the superficial—and often artificial—lives of people all over the world. These days it's incredibly easy to significantly alter your appearance just by opening an app.

CHANGE YOUR MIND INSTEAD OF TRYING TO CHANGE YOUR BODY: PHOTO EDITING AND BODY DYSMORPHIC DISORDER

Photo editing software and those seemingly innocent photo filters can unintentionally contribute to stress, termed "SnapChat Dysmorphia" in scientific literature. This *JAMA* article explains it well:

> We live in an era of edited selfies and ever-evolving standards of beauty. The advent and popularity of image-based social media have put Photoshop and filters in everyone's arsenal. A few swipes on Snapchat

can give your selfie a crown of flowers or puppy ears.
A little adjusting on Facetune can smoothen out skin,
and make teeth look whiter and eyes and lips bigger. A
quick share on Instagram, and the likes and comments
start rolling in. These filters and edits have become
the norm, altering people's perception of beauty
worldwide.

The pervasiveness of these filtered images can take a
toll on one's self esteem, make one feel inadequate for
not looking a certain way in the real world, and may
even act as a trigger and lead to Body Dysmorphic
Disorder (BDD).[25]

Scott here. My first encounter with Body Dysmorphic Disorder
(BDD), an excessive preoccupation with perceived flaws in appearance, came during medical school when I spent several weeks rotating at a high-profile plastic surgeon's office on Michigan Avenue in
downtown Chicago.

I had the opportunity to assist in several rhinoplasties (nose jobs), as
well as face lifts, cheek filling procedures, and many more elective
cosmetic surgeries. I was amazed by the surgeon's ability to match
the image that he and the patient had decided on prior to surgery.

However, I soon realized that for many of his patients, this wasn't
(and would never be) good enough. Even during my short time there,
I saw people coming back in to have a 2nd, 3rd, or 4th nose job, or to
have something else "fixed".

These people would be considered beautiful by most standards, but they simply could not see themselves that way. They were obsessed with any perceived imperfections and wanted them corrected.

Unfortunately, no matter how many surgeries, injections, and other interventions were done, they would never be completely satisfied when comparing themselves to a false standard of physical perfection.

John 3:16 tells us: "For God so loved the world, that he gave his only begotten Son, that whosoever believeth in him should not perish, but have everlasting life."

If you replace the words "the world" with your name, then I think you can start to comprehend your individual worth. If you are worth the incredible price of the life of our Savior, Jesus Christ, why spend your time wallowing in negative self-perceptions?

Apparent limitations and imperfections become meaningless when compared with the love of our all-powerful Father in Heaven.

5 TIPS TO AVOID
THE TRAP OF COMPARISON

1. **REDIRECT**

   We may not even consciously realize that we are comparing our faces or bodies with others. If we are watching out for comparisons that slip into our thought-stream, we can redirect through positive affirmations.

2. **FIND YOUR UNIQUE**

   Find ways to celebrate your God-given talents and characteristics. How boring would life be if we were all the same? Discover what makes you and your spouse different, unique, and special. Take the time to consider how these qualities benefit you and others. How can you use what's unique about you to bless another's life?

3. **MOVE PAST SUPERFICIAL**

   Spend time truly getting to know people instead of assuming that the way they appear online, at church, or in social situations is an accurate and complete representation of them.

4. **FOCUS ON GRATITUDE**

   Writing down what you're grateful for can have a transformative effect on your mindset. It shifts your focus from what is wrong with you and your life to seeing how abundantly blessed you are.

5. **SKIP SOCIAL MEDIA**

   For some it may be necessary to set limits or step completely away from social media. Make an honest assessment of the time you spend and how you feel when you engage in it. If you can't honestly say that it's building you up or providing an opportunity for you to lift others, then find a better use for your time.

Courage to change
the things you can.

NEW HABIT FORMATION

Write down the habit you would like to incorporate, including when you will do it. Whenever possible, pair the desired habit with an existing habit. For situational habits designate an if...then clause.

EXAMPLES

- IF we are tempted to numb in front of the TV after a long day, THEN we will go for a walk or read a book.

- IF we recognize thoughts of comparison, THEN we will recite our positive affirmations and go give somebody a compliment.

_____

_____

_____

_____

_____

_____

_____

_____

_____

_____

_____

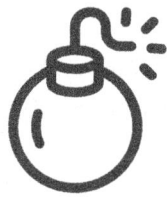

HABIT #3

TAKE BACK CONTROL

Utilize "time-outs"
to clear and refocus
your mind.

TAKE BACK CONTROL

Meditation

There are things in life we just can't change. When those things are causing stress and harming our health, the solution is to change the way our bodies react to stress.

Earlier, we discussed Dr. Rick Hanson's work showing that, although your brain seems to have an inherent negativity bias, it remains plastic (or moldable) throughout your life. This means you can control your brain's response to ongoing stressors by the input you provide.

So, how do we begin to rewire our brains toward a positivity bias rather than a negativity bias? Fortunately, there are several ways to do this:

Meditation, mindfulness, and positivity exercises are powerful tools. Pairing these mental exercises with physical exercise and nature (the next two chapters) can multiply their benefit.

When you choose to step back from stressful situations that you can't control and focus on the positive, you gain control over your outlook and your attitude.

Justin Su'a, Major League Baseball mental performance and leadership coach, advocates taking a personal time-out to look at the bright side. He asks, "When was the last time you took time to pause? Have you ever considered that the speed of life is causing you to feel acted upon instead of remembering that you have the power to act?" [26]

Justin added to that thought in a TEDx talk when he said:

> When the going gets tough, great coaches will call
> a timeout—to regroup the players, to refresh, and
> to help them remember the things that matter most.
> But we don't do that in life. When the deadlines are
> there…you feel like you have to do a little bit more.
> Sometimes trying to go all out leads to burnout, but
> what you needed all along was a time-out.[27]

When you step away from the stress, you tell your brain that the
stressor isn't a threat anymore. Your actions signal to your brain that
it's safe to let the guard down.

Daily Time Outs

We have found that the more frequently you do small activities to
rewire your brain, the greater the benefit. Let's look at what a day of
brain training time-outs might look like:

- 5-10 minutes praying and journaling in the morning.

- 10 minutes sitting outside during your lunch break doing some
  deep breathing and soaking in the sun (preferably with your bare
  feet on the ground.)

- 10 minutes of yoga or stretching before heading to bed.

The key is to do a little bit at a time, consistently. This will be more
beneficial than spending an hour once a week meditating—though
that hour would certainly be better than not doing anything!

Tap into Technology
MEDITATION, MINDFULNESS, AND TECHNOLOGY

For some people, the idea of meditation can be intimidating. For many, it's kind of an obscure (and maybe even weird) practice that feels more at home in a hippy convent or martial arts movie than in your daily routine.

Meditation has its place in those settings, but it is also so much more than that. Meditation can be simply taking the time to be still. Meditation can be prayer and pondering. Meditation can be mental imagery or self-hypnosis.

Technology can make pretty much everything easier, including meditation and mindfulness. There is powerful research showing that you can both measure and affect your stress response by controlling your thoughts.

HEART RATE VARIABILITY

Heart Rate Variability (HRV) is a measurement of the variation in time between each heartbeat. Scientists have discovered that this variation is managed by a part of our nervous system that we don't consciously control, the autonomic nervous system (ANS). The ANS consists of two parts, called the sympathetic (fight or flight) and parasympathetic (rest and digest) systems. These two branches are sending constant signaling throughout the body, including the heart.

If the sympathetic system becomes dominant—because your brain is sensing a stressful situation— then your heart starts beating faster, and the HRV decreases. The opposite is true if you're in a more relaxed state and the parasympathetic nervous system is dominant.

HEART RATE VARIABILITY BIOFEEDBACK (HRVB)

HRVB provides a simple way of measuring your own HRV. You can get live feedback through an app showing how much stress your brain is currently processing. Using the real-time visual, you can learn how to effectively recognize and reverse your body's stress response through relaxation techniques.

SOUND THERAPY

Sound therapy is an intriguing new area of technology that is show-ing some promising results in improving stress response. Binaural beats is a technology that we mentioned in the sleep section (see the 4 Senses of Sleep).

HUSO is another exciting option that we just recently discovered. This promising technology uses enhanced human-based tones that play through headphones and reverberate through pads placed on major acupuncture meridians.

BrainTap is another unique and powerful option in sound therapy. Its goal is to synchronize brainwaves to a specialized sound, consisting of four elements: binaural beats, guided visualization, holographic music (creating the sensation of being completely surrounded by sound), and isochronic tones (which are equal intensity pulses of sound separated by an interval of silence).

NEUROFEEDBACK

Just as we can gain insight into our stress levels through HRV, there are also several tech-related options to do this through a process called Neurofeedback. Neurofeedback often utilizes EEG technology (this is what doctors use to measure brain wave activity) to provide real-time biofeedback.

Some of the tech options available here include the Muse, NeuroSky MindWave and BRAINNO (which simultaneously measures both brain waves and HRV).

MEDITATION APPS

Apps like HeadSpace, The Mindfulness App, Calm, and Mindbody can guide your meditation and help you learn how to do it more effectively. Smiling Mind is an app geared towards children.

More Help

You may find yourself in a situation where you are doing everything that you can to reduce your stress and increase your resilience, but it's still not enough. If you implement the recommendations in this book and find only modest benefits in controlling your stress, anxiety, and depression, then it's time to partner with somebody who can help you.

One of our preferred methods of therapy is called Solution Focused Brief Therapy (SFBT). SFBT is consistent with the way that we work to improve physical and mental health in our practice.

Some forms of therapy are centered around reliving the past. You mentally re-experience traumatic events and stressors in your life with the goal of changing your view of them.

SFBT, in contrast, is all about looking into the future to help you visualize the type of person you want to be and the life you wish to have.

Once you can capture that vision, you stay forward focused, working to make it a reality. You leave the previous trauma, stressors, and baggage behind and strive to keep everything in your life positive and productive.

Dr. Adam Froerer, Associate Program Director, MFT, at Mercer University explains:

> Clients are viewed as agents of change and as the experts of their own lives.
>
> ...despite challenges and previous trauma experiences, clients still have resources they can draw on to cope, and are inherently resilient.
>
> SFBT provides a positive, hopeful, future-oriented approach to trauma treatment that is respectful and guided by strong, resilient and competent trauma survivors![28]

There are also a host of other therapy methods that we have seen provide immense benefit for our patients—from conventional cognitive behavioral therapy, to adventure-based psychotherapy (another favorite of ours!), to hypnotherapy, to energy healing, and more.

We recommend researching any therapist or service provider you are considering. Find out the type of therapy he or she utilizes, areas of interest, and experience.

A visit to see the therapist's office space and requesting a brief consultation may be helpful. You want to make sure that your therapist's techniques, approach, environment, personality, and goals mesh with what you are looking for so you can feel completely comfortable and trust in his or her treatment.

Utilize "time-outs" to clear and refocus your mind.

NEW HABIT FORMATION

Write down the habit you would like to incorporate, including when you will do it. Whenever possible, pair the desired habit with an existing habit. For situational habits designate an if...then clause.

EXAMPLES

- As part of our morning routine, we'll spend 10-15 minutes in quiet meditation and prayer.

- We'll plan a time each day when we can each sit quietly by ourselves for a few minutes.

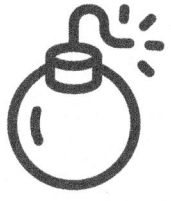

HABIT #4

E X E R C I S E

Moving more means stressing less. Exercise is just as important for mental health as it is for physical health.

EXERCISE

While physical activity significantly reduces your risk of disease, it also has direct benefit in reducing stress.[29] Studies show that this is due to changes in hormone responses, and even changes in certain neurotransmitters (chemical messengers) in the brain—including dopamine and serotonin—that affect mood and behavior.[30]

Exercise can increase our ability to resist the body's typical reaction to stress. In fact, exercise initiates physical change in brain structure and connective pathways between nerve cells.[31] Researchers have also found that being active makes us 43% more likely to experience successful physical, psychological and social aging, as well as better modulation of pain.[32,33,34,35] All of these factors can either contribute to or help mediate stress, making exercise a critical tool for both immediate and long-term stress management.

There are so many ways to exercise.

We have friends and patients who seem to live at the gym and love lifting weights, running on the treadmill, or killing it at CrossFit. If the culture and convenience of working out at a gym helps you be more consistent with your exercise, then that's a huge win.

Outdoor exercise provides a dual benefit by adding in the stress-relieving qualities of being out in nature. Southern Utah is known for a great climate and a huge network of outdoor trails throughout the red rock mountains, so of course there are a lot of avid walkers, runners, cyclists, and mountain bikers here. Not to mention all the golf courses!

Many cities and towns have competitive and leisure sports opportunities for all ages. Find out what people around you are doing. Take a class, join a club, or just show up at the courts for pickup games.

Start Simple

Just start with something. It may be as simple as trying to add more movement into the things you are already doing each day.

Maybe you've heard the campaign that "Sitting is the New Smoking." Whether in driving, working, gaming, or watching, too much time sitting is definitely a plague of the age. Staying mindful of how much you are sitting and working to counteract that can be beneficial to your health and your stress levels.

Some simple changes to help you be more active (and sit less) include:

- Get a standing desk

- Do calf raises while standing at your desk, or while doing the dishes

- Park at the back of the parking lot

- Walk around when you're on the phone

- Have walking meetings

- Walk around your office building during your lunch break

- When working on the computer or watching movies at home, set an alarm to get up every 15-20 minutes

- Do yard work together

- Skip moving walkways, elevators and escalators and take the stairs whenever possible

- Avoid drive-throughs

- Clean your house

- Drink water from a small bottle, so you have to refill it more often

- Carry groceries (when you don't have a lot) in a basket instead of using a cart

- Squeeze a grip strengthener when you're on the phone

- Arrange your office so you have to walk to get to everything (printer, supplies, etc.)

- Plan family activities that encourage movement (wrestling, tag, follow-the-leader, sports, dance, etc.)

Start Slow

Exercise doesn't have to be running or an intense cardio class. Exercise can look different for every person and for every age. While some people might find their optimal stress reset through all-out, exhaustive exercise, others may gravitate more towards the calm-inducing practices that have been a staple of ancient cultures, like yoga and Tai Chi.

We have loved driving by a park in the early morning and seeing the dedication that some of our elderly neighbors have to staying healthy by practicing Tai Chi together with the sunrise. And how amazing is it to see children taught yoga techniques to help them cope with the emotions that a school day can bring?

The stress-reducing benefits of both yoga and Tai Chi have been studied extensively.[36,37,38,39]

Sometimes when we recommend yoga to a patient or friend, the initial response is rejection or even fear. They usually say something like "I'm not nearly flexible enough" or "I'll never be coordinated enough to do yoga."

However, both yoga and Tai Chi are accessible activities for a variety of ages and skill levels. You don't have to be good at it and you don't have to be flexible (Scott)! Like any new skill, you just need to start.

Moving more means stressing less.

NEW HABIT FORMATION

Write down the habit you would like to incorporate, including when you will do it. Whenever possible, pair the desired habit with an existing habit. For situational habits designate an if...then clause.

EXAMPLES

- We'll add yoga or other exercise to our daily morning routine after we finish reading the scriptures.

- We'll discover a new sport and take lessons or join a league that practices weekly.

_____

_____

_____

_____

_____

_____

_____

_____

_____

_____

_____

_____

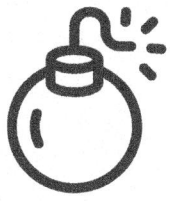

HABIT #5

NATURE

Healing has its roots in nature. Whether physical, mental, emotional, or spiritual, nature heals what ails us.

NATURE

God created the ultimate de-stress mechanism: the great outdoors.

The combination of fresh air, direct physical connection with the earth (grounding), plant life, room to roam, sunlight induced vitamin D and light therapy, beautiful landscapes, birds singing, leaves rustling, starry nights, and circadian rhythm reset somehow brings everything else into perspective.

When we go outside and see how big the world is, we often discover that our problems are smaller than we thought.

Nature delivers peace, comfort, and joy—a robust defense against stress. Research shows that the sun on your face really does make you happy on a biological scale.[40]

Yet, for some reason, the average American spends 93% of their life inside.[41]

We have to make a conscious effort to plan time outside. It is easy to just go about our day, hopping from house-to-car-to-office and back again, five days in a row.

Even starting small, with just a couple of hours a week outside can show measurable results. A recent study of over 20,000 people in England showed that individuals who reported spending at least two hours a week outdoors also reported better physical health and mental wellbeing.[42]

Not only can spending time in nature allow your body and mind to de-stress, it also improves your mood and focus and inspires greater creativity.

A study collecting heart rate and blood pressure data along with self-reported stress levels indicated "that spending time in outdoor environments, particularly those with green space, may reduce the experience of stress, and ultimately improve health." [43]

Sun exposure has immense health benefits, including cancer prevention[44] and lowering blood pressure and risk of heart attack.[45] Sunlight increases your metabolism and might help your jeans fit better.[46] Even just more natural light coming in your windows can provide pain relief and lower stress.[47]

Vitamin D

Vitamin D levels are a critical—and vastly undervalued—indicator of health. While supplements abound, the optimal and most efficient way to increase your vitamin D is through sun exposure. Ultraviolet rays of sunlight soak into our skin and initiate a molecular conversion that is then processed through the liver and kidneys to form bioavailable vitamin D.

Several factors affect how much vitamin D we can gather from time in the sun. The season, time of day, amount of cloud cover (or smog… yuck) can all affect how much vitamin D your body can absorb.

Sunscreen applied specifically or as part of a lotion or makeup product restricts this mechanism.[48]

Contrary to popular belief, where you live on the planet (and how directly overhead the sun is) does not consistently predict vitamin D levels. There is plenty of opportunity for your body to form vitamin D (and store it in the liver and fat) from sunlight during the spring, summer, and fall months, even in the far north latitudes.

If you live in a grayer climate you can still access 50% of the UV energy from the sun through complete cloud cover. Shade and severe pollution will limit you to 40% availability. Even though it feels great to sit by a sunny window, it won't give you any vitamin D—UVB radiation can't travel through glass.[49]

Don't tell your overzealously modest grandma we said this, but it's important that you don't cover up too much when you're trying to increase your vitamin D. You won't get enough sun to show positive change in vitamin D with just intermittent arm and face exposure. If you want to interpret that to mean you should become regulars at the nude beach, that's on you.

We recommend testing your vitamin D regularly. It's an inexpensive lab test and keeping track of your levels can give you more control over your health and performance.

Essential Oils

People have been using essential oils to harness the powerful benefits of nature for centuries and there is a lot of modern research demonstrating specific stress-relieving capabilities.

LAVENDER

Lavender essential oil, in particular, has a pronounced ability to slash stress. In a head-to-head study comparing the treatment of adult anxiety with lavender essential oil versus lorazepam, a common anti-anxiety medication, the lavender was just as effective. Almost all variables

studied, including anxiety, worry, severity of illness and sleep distur-
bance, improved significantly and similarly in both groups. By six
weeks of treatment, the results were even better in the lavender group
compared to the lorazepam group. Not surprisingly, lavender oil has
significantly fewer side effects, has no potential for abuse, and causes
no hangover effects.[50]

Lavender has shown stress-busting benefits when taken orally,[51] dif-
fused into the air,[52] and topically in aromatherapy massage.[53,54]

A peppermint and lavender blend demonstrated positive effect on
anxiety and sport skill performance in one study.[55]

OTHER EXCITING EVIDENCE-BASED OPTIONS
Published research on bergamot essential oil shows that inhalation
can alleviate work-related stress,[56] lower blood pressure and stress
response,[57] and affect mood, nervous system, and cortisol.[58]

A 2006 study involving hospice patients with terminal cancer showed
aroma hand massage with bergamot reduced pain, anxiety, and
depression.[59]

One study measuring the effects of aroma mouthwash showed significantly lower perceived stress in the aroma mouthwash group versus
control and saline groups.[60]

Additional research showed that inhaling an essential oil blend of
lemon, eucalyptus, tea tree, and peppermint had a positive effect on
stress, sleep quality and immunity in healthy adults.[61]

A study comparing the effects of massage with a carrier oil versus carrier oil + roman chamomile essential oil demonstrated that "the addition of an essential oil seems to enhance the effect of massage and to improve physical and psychological symptoms, as well as overall quality of life." [62]

Different studies have shown that sweet orange essential oil alone[63], as well as a blend of lavender, roman chamomile, and neroli[64] essential oils, both show similar benefits in decreasing symptoms of anxiety (which are very similar to the symptoms of a stress response).

Healing has its roots in nature.

NEW HABIT FORMATION

Write down the habit you would like to incorporate, including when you will do it. Whenever possible, pair the desired habit with an existing habit. For situational habits designate an if...then clause.

EXAMPLES

- We'll spend at least part of our lunch time outside each day.

- We'll spend 20 minutes a day gardening or doing yard work.

PURPOSE & COMMITMENT

Once you can define and connect to your deeper meaning and soul purpose, your path becomes clear.

COMMITMENTS, COVENANTS, AND ACCOUNTABILITY

AS WE DISCOVER our deeper purpose and meaning in this life, we must be willing to move toward it.

In the Stress section we discussed how divine discontent drives us to become better, stronger, wiser, and holier. As we recognize the gap between where we are and where we want to be, we rally the motivation to get there. We commit to changing our thoughts and behavior in order to reach the potential we are just beginning to visualize.

Commitments

A critical part of maintaining motivation through the inevitable roadblocks of life is making and keeping commitments.

Think about the most important decisions you've made in your life and the commitments connected to them. Marriage. Raising children. Beginning a graduate or post-graduate training program. Starting a new job or your own business. Accepting a volunteer position in your church or community. When difficulties come up in any of these situations, you make the effort to navigate through them because of your commitment.

Compare those scenarios with quick decisions you've made on a whim, but then later opted not to pursue. When things got hard, you may not have even thought twice about changing directions, because you were never actually committed.

Covenants

In the Church of Jesus Christ of Latter-day Saints, we call commitments made between us and God, covenants. Sometimes these covenants include another person—as with the eternal covenant of marriage.

Making a commitment with another person—and especially with God—creates accountability. For many people, this is the exact reason to avoid commitments. However, couples who strive for greater power and purpose in their lives recognize that commitment and accountability are critical ingredients of change.

Accountability

We believe that the more knowledge we attain in this life, the more accountable we are for the decisions that we make. For example, a child lacks complete comprehension of the purpose behind rules and laws, and thus is not held to as high of a standard as adults when he/she breaks the law.

This can be intimidating and may initially cause one to second guess whether it's worth obtaining advanced knowledge and understanding. However, striving to become our best self-motivates us to keep learning. Why?

Increased opportunities and growth are only possible through increased knowledge and accountability.

Commitments and accountability can become powerful catalysts for change in our lives. The process looks something like this:

1. RECOGNIZE

You recognize that you would like to improve something about yourself—your ability to think and reason more clearly, your energy levels, your physical strength, your capacity to love or forgive, your ability to work well with others, your ability to meet deadlines, your integrity, or your faith.

2. ANALYZE

Write down what you are currently doing in your life to develop this trait, knowledge, or skill. Keep a focus on your deeper meaning as you consider adding potential supporting activities.

NOTE: Some people move through these first two steps and think it is enough. Just deciding you want to change and figuring out how to do it will rarely result in sustainable lifestyle changes.

3. COMMIT

Make a commitment with another person, preferably your spouse. Include Heaven in this commitment. As you make specific plans for how to carry out the necessary changes, you will be held accountable to your spouse and to God.

This may mean that you start your day off with a prayer, stating how you plan to work on your goal that day. This will help you keep your plan in your thoughts throughout the day and help remind you to occasionally pray again about the commitments you made that morning.

As temptations come along to fall back into the same detrimental habits, you find added strength and resolve to keep your commitment, knowing that at the end of the day you'll be reporting both to your spouse and to God.

Each day, your ability to do and become better increases a little. This happens slowly, almost imperceptibly, but it happens.

We'll frequently hear patients tell us of their surprise and delight as they realize that they no longer crave the caffeine and sugar they thought they could never live without. Or, they realize that their energy and brain clarity have increased to the point where they are much more productive at work and still have the energy to play with their kids when they get home. They didn't recognize the incremental improvements, but one day realized that that they were free of the addictions and weaknesses they committed to work on.

Knowing your purpose gives you power. The following five chapters will walk you through discovering your deeper meaning, finding purpose through service, gratitude, and journaling, and taking control of your mindset.

JOHN

JOHN WAS AWARE that his health was declining and made periodic attempts at change, but nothing brought lasting results. By the time he came to us, John was in his late fifties, had aching joints, and felt tired all of the time. He couldn't concentrate at work and had constant sugar cravings. Between his busy job and a demanding volunteer position at church, he was feeling stress.

Blood work confirmed our suspicion of metabolic syndrome. John had elevated insulin levels and blood sugar—above the cutoff for Type 2 Diabetes. He also had elevated triglycerides and LDL cholesterol, high blood pressure, and was overweight, particularly around his midsection.

As we discussed John's results, his initial response was shock and sadness, to the point of tears. All of the emotion and fear involved with his decline in health seemed to become a reality as we explained his situation. As we moved past the diagnosis and started to talk about the root causes of these issues, he began to understand that these were things that he could control. His fear was replaced with determination. He was ready to change!

All that John needed was an understanding of where he was at and specific instructions on how to start. He committed to both me and to his wife that he was ready to make the recommended changes. John later shared with me that he also went home and made a commitment to God. He told me that he realized his physical ailments were affecting his spiritual sensitivity and growth and he knew he needed the Lord's help.

John utilized an app on his watch that allowed him to track his steps, weight, and blood pressure and created competitions and games that motivated him to improve. This allowed him to share his progress easily with me and others and add even more accountability to his commitments.

Within a few weeks, John found that his constant sugar cravings were gone, and his energy levels were improving. He was losing one to three pounds a week—slower than he had hoped, but it was consistent and sustainable weight loss. John's blood pressure normalized after about two months, without ever adding any medications. When we re-tested his labs after three months, John was overjoyed to see that his cholesterol was back to optimal ranges and that he no longer had diabetes.

John's work was far from done, but the evidence of his efforts added fuel to the fire and his progress continues. He has now lost a total of thirty-four pounds, and is more productive at work, at home, and at church.

In the beginning, John was checking in with me weekly to keep himself accountable. Now I only hear from him every few months, because the initially challenging changes have become his everyday habits.

CULTURE OF PURPOSE & COMMITMENT

#1: Discover Your Deeper Meaning
*If you know your "why" then everything
else in life becomes easier.*

#2: Service
*Step outside of yourself by watching for
ways to serve others*

#3: Gratitude
*Gratitude is one of the most powerful tools
for transformation.*

#4: Journaling
*Write your life story both before
and after it happens.*

#5: Mindset
*Expand your mindset with
visualization and positive affirmations.*

HABIT #1

DISCOVER YOUR DEEPER MEANING

If you know your "why" then everything else in life becomes easier.

DISCOVER YOUR
DEEPER MEANING

Deciding to mindfully live your purpose mobilizes the transition from wading in the mud of mediocrity to becoming a high achiever.

It is the difference between being the victim or being the hero in your life.

It is acting instead of reacting.

It is deciding who you are, what drives you, and ultimately, who you want to become.

Once you can define and connect to your deeper meaning and soul purpose, your path becomes clear.

Personal Mission and Vision Statements

A successful business is built on a foundation of a clearly defined mission and vision. A successful business does not allow anything to interfere with its mission. No matter how good a diverging opportunity might be, if it does not align with this purpose it is left behind.

Sometimes we notice that diverging opportunities have begun to creep into our family life. These are almost always good things. The problem is, they are not the best things. We have decided that we need to reserve most of our time for the best things in our lives. If we can't be selective with our time and energy, we will look back and find that we have been lulled into mediocrity instead of maximizing our potential.

Approaching your marriage and your life with the same absolute clarity and daily focus that powers a Fortune 500 company, will ensure enduring personal success.

Crafting personal and family mission and vision statements is a great way to clarify your purpose. Revisiting them frequently will help you keep your activities aligned with your ultimate goals.

In the Church of Jesus Christ of Latter-day Saints, we receive a special blessing called a patriarchal blessing that provides personalized direction from God and shares some of the promises and gifts that we will receive as we live worthy of them. Using this direction as you develop your personal mission statement can be very helpful.

Our own family mission statement has had several revisions over the years, and this is where we have settled:

> As disciples of Jesus Christ, we strive to reflect his gospel and his light. We live with integrity as we carefully follow prophets, honor our covenants, and strive to fulfill our divine potential. We protect the sanctity of our home and live worthy of the constant companionship of the Holy Ghost. As an eternal family, we treat each other with respect, kindness, and love.
>
> We find joy and purpose in working hard, serving others, and developing our skills and talents. We value learning and reading. We are passionate about good food, family, and friends. We continually seek out new adventures and love discovering other cultures.
>
> We make the world around us brighter as we share goodness. "Let your light so shine before men, that they may see your good works, and glorify your Father which is in heaven." *Matthew 5:16*

Recognize, Analyze, and Commit

Science is showing that living your purpose protects your brain and decreases your risk of Alzheimer's by half.[1] Another study followed almost seven thousand adults for four years and found that increased purpose in life (PIL—it's an actual scientific term) leads to a significantly reduced risk of stroke.[2] In a study of 1500 participants with cardiovascular disease, those with increased PIL had a much lower risk of heart attack after two years.[3,4] It's no surprise that having a purpose in life has actually proven to keep you living life longer.[5] It is intriguing to see it broken down into statistics though:

> One study found that a strong sense of purpose was associated with a 72 percent lower rate of death from stroke, a 44 percent lower rate of death from cardiovascular disease, and a 48 percent lower rate of death from any cause in a population of men after an average of thirteen years of follow-up.[6]

In the beginning of this section we talked about the process of recognizing, analyzing, and committing. We're going to apply that to discovering and living your purpose.

1. RECOGNIZE

Begin by keeping track of what you do for one day or reflecting honestly on how you spent your time the day before.

2. ANALYZE

- Write down a list of things that you would want to do if you knew that you had one week to live.

- Now, write down a list of things that you would do if you had one year to live.

Compare and consider how you actually spent the previous day. What about the past week, and the month before that?

Consider your lists and see how many of your "ideal life" things you are doing on a daily, weekly, or monthly basis. If the things on your lists are not showing up in your daily living, you need to realign. The goal of this exercise is to help you reclaim what is really important in your life by making a part of each day.

Rewrite everything that you do during a day under three columns:

1. Essential Activities and Motivation
These are your core values—what you live for. Your dreams and your goals. These are activities that bring you joy.

2. Supporting Activities
Things that must be done to enable essential activities. Work is usually a supporting activity. While our work should be fulfilling, it exists to allow us to provide for our family's needs and as a vehicle for growth, learning, and service.

3. Fluff
Things that don't actually bring you lasting joy and don't empower your essential activities. Things that distract you from relationships, suck up time, and numb you to what is really important.

What percentage of your time is focused on primary and meaningful moments versus supporting activities? Do you work so much that you don't have any time left for living your purpose? How much of your day is simply wasted time?

The way that we allocate time indicates what is most important to us. Matthew 6:21 teaches, "For where your treasure is, there will your heart be also."

Joe J. Christensen elaborates on that, asking: "How do we determine where our treasure is? To do so, we need to evaluate the amount of time, money, and thought we devote to something"[7]

Living with integrity requires that we spend more time on the things that matter more. What do you need to change in your schedule so that it reflects and upholds your core purpose?

3. COMMIT

Now you have a key to the map of your life. You know what is important to you. Your primary activities are **WHERE** you want to go. Your supporting activities are **HOW** you will get there. The fluff is the roadblocks—the things that will prevent you from finding true joy and success.

Commit to:
- Align your daily, weekly, and monthly living with your core values and with what brings you joy

- Maintain a proper balance between essential and supporting activities

- Get rid of the fluff and roadblocks in your life

In the Book of Mormon, two major civilizations (Nephites and Lamanites) were at war. The following verse has a lesson for all of us in determining our motivations:

> Nevertheless, the Nephites were inspired by a better cause, for they were not fighting for monarchy nor power but they were fighting for their homes and their liberties, their wives and their children, and their all, yea, for their rites of worship and their church.[8]

If you want to win at life then, like the Nephites, you need to make sure that what you are fighting for inspires you to give your all.

In a recent article, Ben Hardy said,

> Almost everything is a distraction from what really matters. You really can't put a price-tag on certain things. They are beyond a particular value to you. You'd give up everything, even your life, for those things. Your relationships and personal values don't have a price-tag. And you should never exchange something priceless for a price.[9]

Commit to Your Marriage

Is being a power couple part of your purpose? If so, you need to honor your marriage commitment over lesser commitments you make on this earth. Russell M. Nelson, President of the Church of Jesus Christ of Latter-day Saints, gave the following advice when speaking to a group of men—but it applies equally to women: "Let nothing in life take priority over your wife [or husband]—neither work, recreation, nor hobby."[10]

If you know your "why" then everything else in life becomes easier.

NEW HABIT FORMATION

Write down the habit you would like to incorporate, including when you will do it. Whenever possible, pair the desired habit with an existing habit. For situational habits designate an if...then clause.

EXAMPLES

- We'll recite our family mission statement together every Sunday morning.

- IF we are considering a new commitment, THEN we'll weigh it against our core values and decide what to get rid of to make room.

HABIT #2

SERVICE

Step outside of yourself by watching for ways to serve others

---

SERVICE

How can service help you find your purpose?

Selfless service not only helps you understand yourself better, it helps you make yourself better.

As noted in the introduction, a power couple is a couple who can make a meaningful difference in the world and in the lives of those around them.

There is something beautiful in this process of trying to make a difference in others' lives that actually changes you. You develop a greater sense of gratitude. The struggles, trials, and challenges you face seem less significant as your focus shifts away from yourself to the needs of others. People who serve others report a greater sense of purpose and meaning in their lives.[11]

Religious leader David A. Bednar said,

> Selflessly serving others counteracts the self-centered
> and selfish tendencies of the natural man. We grow
> to love those whom we serve. And because serving
> others is serving God, we grow to love Him and our
> brothers and sisters more deeply. Such love is a mani-
> festation of the spiritual gift of charity, even the pure
> love of Christ.[12]

With each service opportunity you gain energy and excitement for serving again. You realize that the way to make the greatest contribution to your family, community, and the world is to strive to become the best that you can be and help others to do the same.

How to Make Service Part of Your Day

We are constantly surrounded by opportunities to serve, but sometimes we are just so busy that we don't see them. Here are a few service scenarios you may not immediately recognize:

- You're rushing out on your way to work, maybe leaving a few minutes later than you'd like. As you're getting into your car, you see that your neighbor's trash hasn't been taken out to the street and it's trash pick-up day. Instead of rationalizing that your neighbor will surely be out any minute to take it out, and you don't have time to do it, you drop your bag and quickly wheel it to the street.

- As you're walking into the front doors of your office building you see somebody still in the parking lot carrying a load and heading toward the doors. Again, you're in a hurry, and the easy thing to do is rush into your office and start your day. Nobody would expect otherwise with how far behind you this person is trailing. On this occasion, though, you wait the somewhat awkwardly long time for him to make it to the door.

- You and your significant other run to the store just before closing time to grab the last parts needed to finish your weekend project. As you enter, you notice an older couple attempting to load large cabinets into their truck. You don't know if it would be offensive to offer to help, and you know there's a chance that if you help them you may not find what you need inside the store, but you stop and help anyway.

- While attending a block party, you notice a young family that just moved into the neighborhood sitting off to the side by themselves.

Although you see some good friends you'd like to talk to, you instead take the time to meet the new family and help them to feel welcome.

Or these are even more simple ideas, but they can make a huge difference to somebody:

- Look for someone who needs a smile

- Say something kind to somebody you see frequently, but maybe don't recognize regularly

- Send a text to a friend or family member to express gratitude

- Invite a family over for dinner (one of our personal favorites)

- Leave an uplifting comment on somebody's social media post

- Take a few minutes to talk to a neighbor

- Visit an elderly widow or widower in your neighborhood

- Compliment somebody who may not receive a lot of attention

- Remember people's names, birthdays, and other special events

Scott here. Being married to a wife who is always looking around for opportunities to serve has taught me to get outside of my own mind and my own worries, and to see the world around me in a different way. I've gradually started to notice people around me more and more. I've experienced how much richer life can be when it's filled with people you have come to know and love through serving them, serving with them, and inevitably being served by them.

IT'S BEEN MY great privilege to get to know some amazing power couples through my profession. Jack and Susan are one of those couples. Both in their later years now, it's inspiring to hear them talk about the priorities they've set in their lives and how that has directed their paths.

Jack and Susan recognized that service was their joint purpose in life and used it to tie their activities and their lives together—serving their family and their community. Over many years of marriage, Jack and Susan honed the ability to recognize the good in others, focus on the positive, and maintain an enlarged vision and perspective of what life is all about.

As the parents of nine children, they made it a point to serve together, working and playing as a family. Jack and Susan both served the community in their jobs as educators for many years.

As Christians, they dedicated many hours in their younger years to serving in their church and later offered their time and talents in full-time service as missionaries for the Church of Jesus Christ of Latter-day Saints in multiple areas throughout the U.S.

For Jack and Susan, their purpose has been largely driven by their personal beliefs.

As members of the Church of Jesus Christ of Latter-day Saints they, like those in many other faiths, see this life as a small part of a much larger (eternal) existence. As such, they have increased motivation to improve themselves each day and also to build up each other and those around them.

Jack and Susan, of course, have individual personalities, ideas, and talents that make them unique, but they have worked for almost fifty years of marriage to become united in the areas of life they believe matter most.

Step outside of yourself by watching for ways to serve others

NEW HABIT FORMATION

Write down the habit you would like to incorporate, including when you will do it. Whenever possible, pair the desired habit with an existing habit. For situational habits designate an if...then clause.

EXAMPLES

- We'll dedicate time during our daily commute to think of a way to serve somebody that day.

- We'll invite a new family over to play board games each Sunday evening.

HABIT #3

GRATITUDE

Gratitude is one of the
most powerful tools
for transforming your
mindset and your world.

GRATITUDE

Have you ever experienced how gratitude can totally shift your perspective? Living with gratitude has the power to make everything in your life better. And one person living with gratitude can have a profound impact on the people around them.

If you have never heard of the Pollyanna effect, then you have a Friday movie night coming to you. (Yes, you—it has made grown men cry, just embrace it). If a little girl can change a town through sharing her optimism and gratitude, think of how you could change your relationships, your family, and your neighborhood.

Gratitude has a host of physical personal benefits. Research demonstrates that positive emotions can change your heart rate variability, which can be utilized to control stress response. It also has implications in treating hypertension, with researchers suggesting that gratitude could be beneficial in reducing the likelihood of sudden death in individuals with congestive heart failure and coronary artery disease.[13]

Gratitude has the power to upgrade your health and makes you and those around you happier.

Perspective

When you bring gratitude into a situation it's like looking at a tropical storm from a satellite instead of from the beach. Both views are real, but the broader perspective allows you to see the situation from a protected position where you can weather the storm without the total devastation that would be felt on the ground. Through gratitude you can rise above the trials and tribulations of life and view them with the understanding that this too, shall pass.

We've had people with good intentions try to prepare us for the difficulty that sometimes comes with change. People warned that the first year of marriage is difficult as you try to create a new life together. Others would tell us to be ready for having children, because that can really tax a relationship.

When we moved to Chicago for Scott to begin his medical school journey there were some people that complained about the difficulty, the schedule, the incessant study hours, the tests, and of course, the debt. They made it sound and look miserable.

Yet, there were people that made it look easy and even fun.

It was all about their focus and perspective. Those who focused on being grateful for the time that they had together made the most of it. Some of our very best memories are the barbecues, game nights, adventures, and road trips with friends who chose to do their best at school and fill the rest of their lives (even though it was sometimes a small portion of their time) with joy.

It was easy to feel and express gratitude when we thought about our friends who had jobs that require constant travel and especially those who served in the military. Our situation was truly nothing when compared to a friend who was serving overseas in life-threatening circumstances for 18 months—he missed the birth of his baby and the first year of her life.

If we look around, we can always find somebody who appears to have it better than us. However, if we take a second look, we can always find people who are enduring trials that we would never ask for.

Gratitude is perspective, and perspective changes everything.

Gratitude is one of the most powerful tools for transformation.

NEW HABIT FORMATION

Write down the habit you would like to incorporate, including when you will do it. Whenever possible, pair the desired habit with an existing habit. For situational habits designate an if...then clause.

EXAMPLES

- We'll express gratitude daily by dedicating an added portion of our journaling or prayers to gratitude.

- We will set aside a time each day to send a brief thank you note to someone.

_____

_____

_____

_____

_____

_____

_____

_____

_____

_____

_____

_____

HABIT #4

JOURNALING

Write your life story
both before and after
it happens.

JOURNALING

Do you journal? Journaling is becoming a lost art. But it's even more than an art.

Journaling can be therapy, the way that you plan your life, a way to track progress, a way to preserve personal and family memories, a way to be more grateful and purposeful in your daily living, and a vehicle for expanding your mindset.

Keeping a journal can allow you to shift your focus from daily stressors, challenges, and weaknesses to see the extent of your blessings and gifts. Mindful and positive journaling shifts the focus from outside factors to things within your control and empowers you to move beyond the victim mindset.

What Journaling Looks Like

Journaling can be done in so many different ways. It can be a running note kept in your phone or on your computer. You can use a journaling app (bonus: you can set a reminder to write!), or you can hand-write your thoughts in a traditional journal. Some people use Instagram or their personal blog as their journal.

We have been loving The Five-Minute Journal.[14] We both received one as a gift from one of our mentors and have been using them morning and night for the past six months. This practice has made a significant difference in setting up the day for success and evaluating how we can improve for the next day. Our Five-Minute Journals have also been instrumental in increasing our gratitude and awareness of the good things in our lives.

A journal is more than simply a way to document your history, it's also an opportunity to shape your future.

Gratitude Journaling

Take note of the things that benefit your life and express appreciation in your journal. This can be things, people, experiences, and even trials.

A study looking at the association between gratitude and mental and physical well-being reported that "...a conscious focus on blessings may have emotional and interpersonal benefits." [15] Participants in the gratitude outlook groups ended with a greater sense of well-being than comparison groups. This includes an increased ability to experience positive emotions such as enthusiasm and joy and interact with others in positive ways.

Gratitude journaling has scientifically demonstrated improved physical health, showing association with reduced inflammation and improved biomarkers related to congestive heart failure.[16] It's also been shown to calm your mind and help you sleep better.[17]

Writing Down Goals & Visualizing Ideals

A journal is more than simply a way to document your history, it's also an opportunity to shape your future.

Keeping track of your goals as part of your journaling is a significant way to hold yourself accountable. One of the secrets to supercharging your success is to take goal-writing a step further and put down a detailed description of what achieving your goal actually looks like. This can include drawing pictures or pasting in photos. Describe what success looks like to you as specifically and vividly as you can.

Earlier in the book we mentioned Solution Focused Brief Therapy (SFBT). SFBT transforms individuals by helping them visualize how they want their life to be instead of focusing on past addictions, trauma, and abuse. Dr. Adam Froerer, a pioneering expert in SFBT, describes the process, saying:

> Because of this positive view of clients, SFBT clinicians help their clients to describe their preferred future **in great detail** rather than focusing on their deficits and unhealthy coping strategies. This also means that clients are not asked to retell or re-experience their trauma experience by focusing on the terrible events, negative thoughts, and problem behaviors.[18]

You can apply the evidenced-backed principles of Solution Focused Brief Therapy in your journaling and unlock great healing and growth potential. Make your journal be just as much about what you want to happen, as what already did happen.

Document your history

It is important to be real and keep an accurate history, but don't put inordinate focus on negative experiences when you write about what has happened in your life. Choose to see and share more good than bad. If you document the lessons you learn from difficult experiences it turns them into a win—and valuable knowledge for future generations that read your words!

Write your life story both before
and after it happens.

NEW HABIT FORMATION
Write down the habit you would like to incorporate, including when you will do it. Whenever possible, pair the desired habit with an existing habit. For situational habits designate an if...then clause.

EXAMPLES

- We'll spend 30 minutes writing in our journals on Sundays after church.

- Each Friday we'll dictate the memories we want to record from the week as we're driving home from work.

HABIT #5

MINDSET

Expand your mindset with high-performance secrets like visualization and positive affirmations.

MINDSET

Proverbs 23:7 teaches, "For as he thinketh in his heart, so is he".

Do you believe that to be true? That our thoughts determine who we are—and who we can become?

Scott here. Have you ever been challenged to do something you didn't think that you could do? I have. And the fact that somebody believed in me enough to even consider challenging me expanded my mindset and changed my life.

And actually, it was three people in particular.

As a teenage boy who lived and breathed basketball, swimming, and skateboarding, I didn't spend a lot of time thinking about much else— and especially not my future.

But because I loved sports, during my last year of high school, I took a sports medicine course at the nearby community college and worked as an aid in a physical therapy office. I loved learning how the body works, and I thought it would be amazing to be a physical thera- pist, but I wasn't sure that I had the grades or stamina to get into—or get through—a physical therapy program.

One day after English class, my favorite teacher, Mrs. Cross, asked me what I wanted to do with my life. I told her that I loved health and that I liked my job in the physical therapy office, so maybe I would try to do something in that field.

She then said something that I had never even considered. Something along the lines of, "Well, if you love health, you could also consider going to medical school and becoming a doctor!" The way she said it made it sound as though it could actually happen. My first inclination was to just brush it off—that was not even within my realm of possibilities at that point in my life.

I did one year's worth of classes at the local university before leaving for a two-year mission for my church to Detroit, Michigan. I learned to speak Spanish and a lot about myself during those two years. I returned home with my world and my mindset greatly expanded.

Shortly before I boarded a plane to go back home, I was able to spend some time with one of the most influential mentors I have had and the President of the Detroit, Michigan mission, Alvin Emery.

During our conversation, he asked me a big question: "If you could dream big and be anything you wanted to be, what would your dream job be?" I admitted to him that I had always been intrigued by the way the brain works and thought it would be amazing to be a neurosurgeon.

My memory has never let go of his firm, booming reply: "In the last two years you have learned a new language. You have learned how to apply yourself in study and how to lead others. You've gained important social skills and confidence in many other areas. You should realize that you can now do whatever you want to do."

As I returned home and found myself at the apex of life's biggest decisions, I kept considering those words. I prayed and pondered on the possibilities, seeking some confirmation that if I was brave enough to embark on that long and incredibly intense journey, that I wouldn't be doing it on my own.

As I was pondering neurosurgery as a real consideration, I talked to a mentor who was a physician. His encouragement, combined with the confirming feelings of the Spirit, helped me to have the courage to move forward and apply to the undergrad Neuroscience program at Brigham Young University and then later submit applications to medical schools across the country.

Several years later, my neurosurgery and neurology rotations in downtown Chicago confirmed to me how much I loved learning about the brain. However, I realized that, like the other specialties I was rotating through, it was only one piece of the puzzle. Ultimately, I felt strongly that the best fit for me was in Primary Care where I could have a broader reach and help to prevent the problems I was seeing.

A few key people in my life challenging me to consider medicine as a career and expressing their confidence in me, opened the possibility of going beyond what I ever thought I could do.

Thinking Big

How many people don't try something because it's not even within their realm of possibilities?

How many people achieve astounding feats because they think it is possible and do the work to make it happen? The only difference is how big they are willing to think.

Our thoughts can limit us, or they can free us.

Oprah Winfrey once said, "Create the highest, grandest vision possible for your life, because you become what you believe."

A fascinating study done in 2007 illustrates the power our thoughts can have on physical outcomes:

Female housekeepers working in a hotel were given physical assessments and then randomly divided into two groups. One group was provided specific examples demonstrating that their work, cleaning hotel rooms, was good exercise. Reports collected after four weeks showed that the women in the informed group felt that they were getting a lot more exercise than they were before and another physical assessment revealed that "they showed a decrease in weight, blood pressure, body fat, waist-to-hip ratio, and body mass index." [19]

Nothing changed for these women except their mindset. Both groups were still doing the same amount of work, but the participants that thought of their work as "exercise" exhibited actual physical change.

You might be thinking, "Well, wouldn't that be great if somebody could just trick me into losing weight?" That would be awesome—but what is even more awesome is recognizing how much power we can have over our lives if we can harness the power of our thoughts.

The power of placebo is amazing, but it requires a naive victim. If we choose a "creator" mindset over a "victim" mindset, then we can take action and take control. There's this interesting cycle where we can change our thoughts by changing our actions and then our thoughts change our actions and our outcomes. Here's an example:

- **YOU CHANGE YOUR ACTIONS:**
  At morning, noon, and night you write, read, and say a positive affirmation, stating that you are confident enough to take on only the most significant and essential projects at work.

- **THOSE ACTIONS CHANGE YOUR THOUGHTS:**
  When a request comes up, you weigh it against the positive affirmation that is still present in your mind and find it lacking.

- **THOSE THOUGHTS CHANGE YOUR ACTIONS:**
  You are confident enough to turn down the request so you can focus on priorities.

- **THOSE ACTIONS CHANGE YOUR OUTCOMES:**
  You are much more productive and successful at work because you are only focusing on what you do best. Doing your best work all the time delivers more confidence into your life.

Circumstances Determine Mindset...Sometimes

Your mindset is highly defined by your circumstances and many people never rise above that.

Those who accomplish the extraordinary figure out how to make their own "get out of jail free" card. They break down the walls in their head imposed by social class, familial upbringing, and neighborhood.

Some of the greatest stories ever told involve a surprising ascent to fame, glory, or power. We are fascinated with rags-to-riches stories, thrilled to find an unlikely hero rising out of the ashes.

But do we think that is possible for ourselves?

How often do you consider the possibility that you can move beyond the limits prescribed for you? If you didn't answer "daily," then broadening your mindset is going to make a big difference in your life.

As you begin to recognize the power of an expanded mindset you unlock the door to a world of possibilities.

Talents are Great; Determination is Critical

Have you ever met somebody who doesn't have any talents? We haven't either.

There may be people who suppress their talents, but we believe that everybody has God-given traits and natural skills that they can work with and mold as they desire. So, identify your talents, pull up your bootstraps, and get to work.

TIP: If you're not sure what your talents are, ask the positive people in your life. They know what you are good at and they'll be happy to tell you.

Recognize that success is primarily about determination. Being good at something is important, but talent means nothing without hard work. If you can allow yourself to dream big and believe that you are capable of everything that it will take to get you there, then wow—the possibilities become endless!

The Power of Positivity

Understanding the power of mindset often begins with recognizing what drives people. It's the difference between individuals who live with gratitude versus people entrenched in a victim mindset and filled with negativity.

We all have examples of both types of people in our lives—and probably most of us have stories of how shifting our sphere of influence to include more positive people, and less negative energy, makes us happier. We should be constantly striving to surround ourselves with people who lift us up, just as we should be seeking to be someone that lifts others.

There has been much written about developing a growth mindset and living with abundance versus scarcity. These are valuable areas of focus as you learn more about mindset and as you seek a path to success in business and life. Adjusting your thinking affects everything that you do and how you respond to each situation. It opens the doors for collaboration and exponential growth as a result of combined mental and physical resources.

Positive Affirmations

An incredibly effective way to shift your mindset to be more positive and growth-oriented is through utilizing positive affirmations.

Positive affirmations are most powerful when they are aligned with your core values and deeper meaning. Affirmations should be in first person, present or future tense, and in positive terminology. You can write the same affirmation every day or you can craft new ones daily. Both techniques are powerful. Some examples are:

- I contribute to the world by sharing my talents, skills, and knowledge with others.

- I eat well, prioritize sleep, and exercise to enjoy good health.

- I can accomplish anything I set my mind to.

- I look for the best in others and in every situation.

- I control my feelings and how I choose to respond to others.

- I am a patient and loving spouse and parent.

Research shows that positive affirmations can produce physical and mental benefit, including decreased stress, increased sense of well-being and improved academic performance. In addition, brain-imaging shows actual physical changes in the brain and subsequent behavior changes with future-tense affirmations.[20]

Visualize Daily

Visualizing is a tool used by high achievers in every arena but honed to perfection by Olympic athletes and professional sports teams.

An article in *Psychology Today*[21] highlights research that uses brain imaging to demonstrate that mental training is almost as effective as physical training—even activating the same brain patterns as physical practice. An intriguing study by exercise psychologist, Guang Yue, compared individuals who lifted weights at the gym with people that did mental workouts at home visualizing weight training in their minds. The astounding results showed that while the gym-goers had a 30% average muscle increase, the mental exercise group posted gains of 13.5% without ever lifting a weight!

Athletes mentally train by visualizing a perfect performance over and over. They imagine themselves going through each step and overcoming any potential roadblocks—all the way through to success. You can increase your odds of success (along with your muscle mass, apparently) by incorporating this practice into your daily habits. Visualize the perfect presentation, how you want your business lunch to go, or a positive outcome to a potentially confrontational situation.

Mental & Physical Creation

Steven Covey teaches in The 7 Habits of Highly Effective People that visualization is a foundational pattern in life. Everything is created mentally before it is created physically. He shares the example of the mental and physical creation involved in building a house. A building goes through an extremely detailed and thorough mental creation before you ever pick up a hammer to commence the physical creation.

This truly is the pattern of all things including, we believe, the very world we live in. President Russell M. Nelson instructed:

> Each phase of the Creation was well planned before it was accomplished. Scripture tells us that "the Lord God, created all things ... spiritually, before they were naturally upon the face of the earth.' [22]

We have the power to mentally create our lives before we physically create them. How often do we take advantage of this power and how often do we sit back and allow circumstances or other people to create our lives for us? If we want to be truly successful in any area, we need to proactively design our blueprint for victory and then take every step outlined to make it happen.

Mindset & Marriage

When we were married, the officiator gave Scott the advice to treat Amy like a queen. We were directed to always treat each other as the person that we could become once we reach our full potential.

Our relationships can thrive when we expand our mindset to see our spouse as who they can and will become, rather than just always focusing on present capabilities and restrictions.

When we search for the divine in ourselves and in those around us— especially those closest to us —then we will elevate the way we act, feel, and live.

Expand your mindset with visualization and positive affirmations.

NEW HABIT FORMATION

Write down the habit you would like to incorporate, including when you will do it. Whenever possible, pair the desired habit with an existing habit. For situational habits designate an if...then clause.

EXAMPLES

- We'll read or recite personal positive affirmations in the mirror after brushing our teeth.

- Write a positive affirmation in my journal each morning.

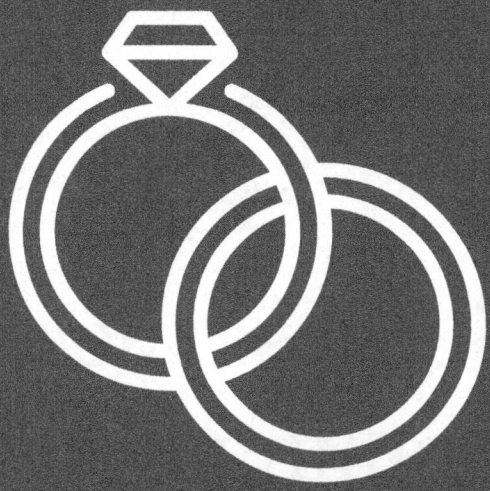

SECTION 5

RELATIONSHIP

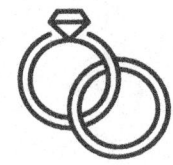

Success means
nothing if you
can't share it
with people that
you love.

BETTER TOGETHER

THE HARVARD STUDY OF ADULT DEVELOPMENT finds that relationships appear to play a major role in developing and maintaining good health.[1] The study began in 1938 and is an ongoing analysis of more than 700 men beginning in their teenage years.

The current director of the study, Dr. Robert Waldinger, and his team have found that people who are more socially connected to family, friends, and community live to be happier and healthier. They also live longer than people who are not as well connected.

In contrast, people who live more isolated lives are less happy and experience a decline in health and brain function earlier in life.

Not surprisingly, the quality of relationships matters as well. Positive relationships appear to be health protective, while living with confrontation—like in a high-conflict marriage—is bad for your health.

Dr. Waldinger points out that people in the study who were most satisfied in their relationships at age 50 were the healthiest at age 80. Even on the days when they experienced more physical pain, they still reported positive mood. Their memories also stayed sharper longer, in contrast with participants who felt that they couldn't depend on their partner and experienced early memory decline.

Does it surprise you that your relationships are just as important to your health as diet and exercise?

A two-decade long research study found that teens who are socially isolated face the same risk for developing inflammation as those who don't exercise and that older adults are more at risk for developing hypertension (high blood pressure) from social isolation than diabetes! Social strain increased the odds of abdominal obesity and inflammation during early to mid-adult years—and carried an even higher risk of overall obesity in older adults.[2]

All of the habits that we have talked about up to this section are critical for optimizing your mental, physical, and spiritual health. Mastering your nutrition, sleep, and stress will help you level up in all areas of your life. But let's be honest, you're not taking your business or your money with you when you die. Your fit and healthy body is staying behind too.

But your relationships—well, those are more than just the here and now. We believe that relationships endure forever.

So, yes, you want to live the best life that you can, perform at your highest capacity, and attain next-level success. But there is a reason we saved this chapter for last:

Success means nothing if you can't share it with people you love.

Relationships are everything.

Utilizing the power of your relationship to improve your nutrition, sleep, stress-management and purpose is one of the great secrets to not only finding success, but also to finding satisfaction in your success.

As you've been working together on the previous sections, we hope that your relationship has also grown. We'd like to build on this growth with five challenges directly targeted at strengthening your relationship. The following chapters focus on communication, selflessness, traditions, individual & mutual growth, and goals.

Research suggests that your relationships are just as important to your health as diet and exercise.

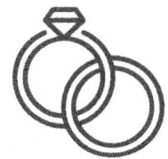

RELATIONSHIP CULTURE

#1: Make Communication Matter
Be clear about needs, celebrate wins together,
and, above all else, choose positivity.

#2: Build a Culture of Selflessness
Look for ways to make your spouse
happy every single day.

#3: Traditions & Memories
Celebrate where you come from and build new
traditions that make the future more exciting.

#4: Foster Individual & Mutual Growth
All growth depends upon activity.

#5: Work Together Towards Goals
Make and review couple and family goals
and help each other be accountable.

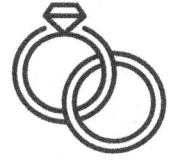

HABIT #1

MAKE COMMUNICATION MATTER

Be clear about needs, celebrate wins together, and, above all else, choose positivity.

MAKE COMMUNICATION MATTER

Communication is just as critical in a relationship as it is in a career.

Just like in a business, you need to be clear about needs, expectations, and goals in order to be united in your direction. Recognition and positive feedback are vital for morale and growth in both business and marriage.

Appreciation is a "relationship booster," with research showing that expressing gratitude predicted next day increase in both relationship satisfaction and connection.[3]

One study concluded that expressing positive emotions is a primary factor in both initiating and sustaining relationships. What the study termed "other-praising" (including showing appreciation and gratitude) is described as the hook that draws potential partners into a relationship and holds relationships together. The research also noted that both partners reported feeling happier and more loving when one expressed positive emotion.[4]

State Needs, Solicit Recognition
Simply hoping or expecting that your spouse will guess what you want or that you need affirmation doesn't work.

We made a goal from the very beginning of our relationship to always be upfront with each other about what we want and need. If one of us accomplishes something awesome, we come home and say, "Look what I did today!" instead of waiting around for the spouse to notice. Sometimes that means saying "No children died on my watch today" and we celebrate appropriately.

A study of 79 dating couples showed that couples who responded enthusiastically to each other's positive news were more likely to have high quality relationships two months later. Celebrating wins together makes your relationship stronger.[5]

Interestingly, responses to positive news was a stronger indicator than responses to negative news. In other words, communicating well about what went right is more important than talking about what went wrong. Sharing with your spouse, truly listening when he/she shares, and focusing on the positive matters!

No Regrets

Another thing that power couples avoid is using language or saying things that they will regret later. It's critical to learn to control your emotions and your temper. Once trust is damaged it is difficult to repair.

Always keep in mind that the person that you are communicating with is somebody that you love and respect. Even if you are frustrated, it's imperative to stifle negative remarks in the moment. Part of the key to healthy communication is to learn when to stop talking.

Power couples don't threaten each other with divorce. It's just not an option for a power couple. Threats are a show of inner weakness that translates into a weak relationship.

We all make mistakes and sometimes we just say and do things that can be misinterpreted. Sometimes we speak before we fully understand the situation.

When disagreements arise, the way that we deal with them is important.

Research shows that daily communication and healthy conflict resolution result in higher marital quality, but the reverse is not necessarily true. Higher marital quality does not always predict daily communication or conflict resolution.[6]

This means that we can't just assume that if our relationship is good, we don't need to worry about resolving conflict and communicating.

If you aren't mindful about spending time talking with your spouse and fixing problems quickly, your relationship will suffer.

Working together to improve your conflict resolution skills not only improves your relationship, it also reduces stress by lowering cortisol levels.[7]

Be clear about needs, celebrate wins together, and, above all else, choose positivity.

NEW HABIT FORMATION

Write down the habit you would like to incorporate, including when you will do it. Whenever possible, pair the desired habit with an existing habit. For situational habits designate an if...then clause.

EXAMPLES

- IF I did something I am happy about, THEN I will tell my spouse about it instead of waiting for him/her to ask or notice.

- IF I feel my frustration level rising, THEN I will say that I need to go get a drink of water before continuing the conversation.

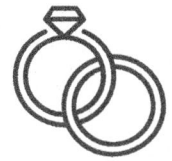

HABIT #2

BUILD A CULTURE OF SELFLESSNESS

Look for ways to make
your spouse happy
every single day.

BUILD A CULTURE OF SELFLESSNESS

Lose Yourself

We have some good friends, Sara and German, who have cultivated a culture of selflessness in their own lives and for their family. They are heavily involved in serving refugees and their local immigrant population, dedicating hours every week to help some of the most underserved individuals in their community.

One year, after we had been friends for a while, German learned how to use a friend's letterpress to make a gift for Sara. He had to practice getting it right, so he shared one of his imperfect attempts with us. This gift has stayed by our bedside for the past 13 years, reminding us what our relationship should be. It reads:

> Husbands, love your wives, even as Christ also loved
> the church, and gave himself for it;
> Ephesians 5:25

When we consider how Christ gave everything for us, even giving up his own life, how does our marriage compare?

If a husband should love his wife so much that he would give his life for her, then does that mean that he should also be willing to give up a basketball game to stay with the kids while she runs errands? Or that he could give up some sleep to help make breakfast for the family in the mornings?

If a wife loves her husband like Christ loves the church, what would that look like?

Would that mean choosing to help her husband prepare for a meeting instead of taking off for a well-deserved girls' night out? Or waking up early to make a lunch for him to take into the office on a busy day?

To Love

Aristotle is credited with saying that happiness and fulfillment is found "by loving rather than in being loved." Selflessness and service is love in action.

One of our great religious leaders, President Gordon B. Hinckley, taught:

> If every husband and every wife would constantly do whatever might be possible to ensure the comfort and happiness of his or her companion, there would be very little, if any, divorce. Argument would never be heard. Accusations would never be leveled. Angry explosions would not occur. Rather, love and concern would replace abuse and meanness...[8]

A lot of us, because of our own family backgrounds, just expect that there will be fighting and arguments in marriage. This is where Power Couples step outside of that expectation and set a new expectation for themselves.

Although we can't be perfect in our relationship, we can strive for an ideal. Having differences of opinion is inevitable—what matters is the way we disagree and how willingly we find a compromise.

Early in our marriage, I (Scott) learned something from Gordon B. Hinckley that has stayed with me. Speaking of his recently departed wife, he said that he had "no recollection of ever having a quarrel with her." [9]

I remember thinking to myself "I don't think I have ever met another couple like that." I rededicated myself to trying to uphold that expectation in our marriage and, despite many other failings along the way, we have been successful in that aspect and it has been an incredible blessing for us.

The more that you think about and try to fulfill the needs of your spouse, rather than your own, the more that your spouse naturally wants to do the same for you. You develop a cycle of always wanting to do the best for each other.

Even though there are small sacrifices along the way, ultimately, both of your needs are always fulfilled, and you can live with gratitude, realizing that your spouse is always caring about you and your needs.

In fact, a study done in 2010 concluded that focusing on other's needs actually ends up making us feel as though our own basic psychological needs are met. Specifically, our needs for autonomy, competence, and relatedness.[10]

This is a very familiar concept in Christianity, as well as other major religions. It's well documented that people who focus less on themselves are happier.

Selfishness or self-centered living can be found at the root of almost all interpersonal and cultural problems.

As documented in Matthew 16:24-25, Jesus Christ taught that

"...If any man will come after me, let him deny himself, and take up his cross, and follow me. For whosoever will save his life shall lose it: and whosoever will lose his life for my sake shall find it."

Deny your "self." Lose your life to find it. Ironic and counterintuitive, but pure truth.

A relationship built on selflessness is the epitome of win-win situations. You find more joy in thinking less about your own needs and desires and more about your spouse and are rewarded with a companion who wants to do everything that they can to make you happy.

Could there be a happier situation?

MICHAEL AND SHIRLEY had been to every kind of doctor imaginable. Their last stop before coming to see us was the Mayo Clinic.

Michael was suffering through a never-ending list of diagnoses, symptoms, prescriptions, and side effects. Shirley was a constant caregiver, unable to leave him for anything more than a quick trip to the grocery store. As I worked with them, I was struck by how much they had been through in the past few years and how much love and effort Shirley put into helping Michael.

In considering what to share in this chapter, I thought of Shirley and asked her to contribute some thoughts for this book describing their relationship and the process that brought her to that hallowed point of nearly perfect selflessness that I observed. I want to synthesize some of the wisdom that Shirley shared, along with some parts of their long and beautiful story together.

In the busy years of raising a family, Michael and Shirley's relationship sometimes took the backseat to other "necessary" priorities. However, they set aside regular time together and overcame difficulties with the knowledge that they had made an eternal covenant and not just an earthly commitment. They kept their focus on God, their relationship, and their family—above all other interests and friendships.

Michael and Shirley had no forewarning of the insurmountable health problems coming their way, but Shirley was able to handle the storm because of habits that she had been prompted to cultivate in the years before, including:

- ▶ Embarking on a deep study to learn how to make her marriage more meaningful

- ▶ Starting a notebook with quotes and personal inspiration about marriage

- ▶ Reviewing her notebook daily—this habit helped renew her resolve in her role as a caregiver

- ▶ Working with a life coach to formulate an ideal life plan

- ▶ Setting goals and priorities that supported that plan, including:

  - To achieve a "celestial, sanctified marriage"

  - To live life without regret, especially regarding her husband

  - To be united in their marriage

Shirley shared so much wisdom and insight with me about how striving for selflessness in a relationship creates a deep and abiding love that can withstand every challenge. She learned these lessons in the midst of endless ER visits, countless tests and procedures, traveling around the country to different doctors, and lying awake at night wishing that there was something she could do to help with Michael's pain.

The following are her own words:

Next to my Heavenly Father, I needed and wanted to put my husband first in my life, even above my children and grandchildren. I made the decision that my marriage would be better than that of my parents and my ancestors. As I prayed, I received answers that I was to be a comfort and inspiration to my husband. Heavenly Father explicitly cautioned me not to be critical of him, but to strive to see him as He sees him and treat him accordingly.

It has been a challenge to break the cultural traditions and habits I learned in my family. I began to pray to see the "God" or good in him and to have the pure love of Christ in my thoughts, words and actions. I made a chart listing all of my husband's virtues and tried to forget any vices. I started keeping a gratitude journal specifically for things I was grateful for in my husband.

I learned that love is dependent on gratitude and that love is more of a decision than an emotion.

I started focusing on my own weaknesses and concentrating on changing myself. To be rid of self-righteousness and judgment was my greatest desire. Slowly, my negative thoughts disappeared, and my life was filled with gratitude and appreciation, not only for my husband, but everyone else around me as well. I was not a negative person overall, but my occasional critical thoughts and words had a detrimental effect on our marriage.

I am not the patient, nurse-like person that many women are. My attitude has been "let's fix it and get on with life." I had to learn how to minister to my husband, whom I loved dearly. It was not a natural or easy thing for me to learn.

I realized that whatever Michael was feeling, I needed to acknowledge and validate. I soon found that the more I did that, the less physical and emotional pain he experienced, because he didn't have to spend time or energy convincing me. This simple principle changed our relationship into a reciprocal and empathetic one and instilled a newfound respect for each other's feelings.

When asked about the time and effort spent in our endless search for help and how that affected me, I can only respond that his life and comfort were everything to me. In something I had read many years ago (one of the notes I reviewed monthly) it mentioned how we should be anxiously concerned for the welfare of our spouse. That took on a whole new meaning for me, as I suddenly was in the middle of 24/7 concern for his welfare.

Not only did I want him to be healed, but when that didn't happen month after month and the prognosis seemed to greatly dim, I wanted him to feel comfort even if he couldn't be healed, especially when he was in so much pain.

Days were spent caring for his needs and when he retired to bed early, I would [stay up late] researching and praying to know what else we could do. My projects, hobbies, and socializing were gladly put on hold. His care was a quest for me—not a burden—to help relieve his suffering and to instill hope for us both. I had to know that I was doing all I could.

Jeffrey Holland said, "True love blooms when we care more about another person than we care about ourselves."[11] I think our true love is blooming. It is my prayer it never stops.

Look for ways to make your spouse happy every single day.

NEW HABIT FORMATION

Write down the habit you would like to incorporate, including when you will do it. Whenever possible, pair the desired habit with an existing habit. For situational habits designate an if...then clause.

EXAMPLES

- Every morning I will make the bed so that our bedroom feels clean and calm when my spouse comes back in.

- I'll text my spouse each day during a break to let him/her know I am thinking about them.

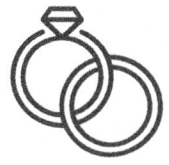

HABIT #3

TRADITIONS & MEMORIES

Celebrate where you come from and build new traditions that make the future more exciting.

TRADITIONS & MEMORIES

What is a tradition? The word can mean different things to different people, but for us it means two things:

1. Remembering: Celebrating our heritage and honoring those who came before us.

2. New Memories: Establishing recurring activities that invite joy into our lives.

Remember Your Heritage

There is something about knowing and honoring your heritage that builds an incredible bond in a couple and family. When you marry and have the opportunity to add to your culture, life gets that much more fun.

Couples who celebrate where they came from have a stronger foundation on which to build new memories and traditions. Learning about each other's backgrounds helps to weave your lives together and builds confidence in your relationship.

In Lori Qian's memoir, *How Sweet the Bitter Soup*,[12] she shares how she and her husband, William, established their marriage on a foundation of two different cultures. They met and fell in love in China before marrying and moving to the U.S. With a Chinese heritage on one side and an American heritage on the other, they wanted to make sure that both histories were represented in their family life. Meeting in the middle meant that each of them had to be willing to move away from some of their childhood traditions and bring the best of both worlds to their new hybrid family culture.

Lori and William wanted to extend the strength of their traditions to their children. They decided to move back to China for a few years to allow the children to experience their rich heritage. In an interview[13] Lori shared:

> [Living in China] gave the kids a really good sense of their identity and an open-mindedness that is so incredibly valuable. William has a very unique background, so trips to the countryside and his hometown gave the kids a different perspective early in life. It strengthened us to be close enough to William's family that we could take part in their annual traditions and travel to his hometown for Chinese New Year.
>
> All those beautiful traditions centered around the concept of "out with the old and in with the new"—cleaning the house, new haircuts, new clothes, and a fresh start—are really special to us now.

The Qians recently moved back to the U.S. after ten years in China. They've gained the strength that comes with knowing and honoring their heritage. They've also gained confidence from making their own way and establishing new family traditions. In Lori's own words:

> Traditions remind us that there's something bigger than what's going on in the moment. That can be so valuable—especially when things are hard. It gives us a lifeline and a broader perspective. It shows us that we are building something.

Make New Memories

Creating new traditions in your relationship provides you with shared hope and anticipation that can carry you through difficult times. Traditions you build as a couple can expand to your children and bring joy to your family relationships. Establishing a framework of fun for your family can be achieved in so many ways.

ADVENTURES

While most of our traditions seem to be centered around food (and we already shared some of those in the Nutrition section), one of our favorite new traditions is "Adventure Saturdays". We try to complete our chores throughout the week so that we can spend afternoons on Saturdays exploring.

We live in a city surrounded by hundreds of hiking trails and we try to take advantage of it! This makes our kids look forward to Saturdays and builds memories that we will forever be grateful for.

GAMES

We decided early on in our marriage that we wanted to adopt a tradition of playing board games together after seeing how close our friend Cade's family was. Cade told how he and his sister often preferred to invite their friends to their house on weekends instead of going out—they had a family tradition of weekend game nights that they didn't want to miss!

When we had the privilege of staying with their family during a trip to Arizona, we were thrilled to be welcomed into their game nights. We have seen our family become stronger through this tradition, just like we saw in their family.

VACATIONS

Some people love to plan trips and travel together—it brings them joy and draws them closer when they experience something brand new together. Amy's brother, Jeff, and his wife, Katy, have built a solid relationship of love, trust, and adventure through their travels around the world.

They fill the walls of their home with photos from their travels and it brings back the joy and thrill of the adventures they shared.

One of our favorite patients, Janet, used to love to go to Hawaii each year with her husband. However, as life got busy and she started having health problems, their tradition got pushed aside.

We started working together on her health and, between nutrition and lifestyle changes and a personalized supplement plan, we were able to wean her off all antidepressants and other medications. Despite this progress, we weren't quite to our goal of having her back to where she was before the health problems started. We tried a few things, but she had plateaued, and we weren't sure why.

Janet and her husband decided that they would reinstate their tradition and plan a trip to Hawaii to celebrate Janet's success in getting off her medications. This was the missing piece. Whatever it was—the stress-relieving sand and sun, the extra vitamin D, or something else entirely—she returned feeling years younger and has been able to maintain her health at that level ever since.

Sometimes traditions can heal not just our spirits, but also our bodies.

HOLIDAYS

Sid, the husband and father of another family that we love, started a yearly tradition with his kids of sending his wife to an exotic location each year for Mother's Day... without ever leaving home. They would decorate the house, dress up, and have food and music that supported the magical illusion. While I'm sure that this amazing wife and mother enjoys a real trip every once in a while, this tradition was one of her yearly highlights and she wouldn't give it up for the world (literally)!

The best memories we carry with us are the fun times we have together. Those memories mean so much more than all the material things we accumulate.

Memories are also among the best gifts that we can give each other. In fact, a study published in 2016 showed that giving experiences builds relationships more than giving objects (even when the experience isn't together).[14]

Traditions Support Family Life

It's important to be willing to be flexible and adapt traditions over time as your family's needs change. If a tradition causes stress or friction, then it becomes a negative factor and needs to be replaced.

Tradition can be doing the same thing at the same place at the same time each year, or it can be taking turns surprising each other with totally new and different things. Traditions make holidays more fun[15] and seasons more exciting. Traditions build stronger relationships and connections, solidify a sense of identity, and add meaning to your life.[16]

Celebrate where you come from and build new traditions that make the future more exciting.

NEW HABIT FORMATION

Write down the habit you would like to incorporate, including when you will do it. Whenever possible, pair the desired habit with an existing habit. For situational habits designate an if...then clause.

EXAMPLES

- Make Friday nights family game night.

- Alternate years to plan surprise anniversary dates or getaways.

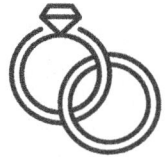

HABIT #4

FOSTER INDIVIDUAL & MUTUAL GROWTH

All growth depends upon activity. There is no development physically or intellectually without effort, and effort means work.

- Calvin Coolidge

FOSTER INDIVIDUAL
AND MUTUAL GROWTH

Individual Growth

While it is important to develop hobbies and traditions together, it is also important to find time to foster your individual growth. Take personal time to learn, practice, and progress while making every effort to support your spouse in his/her endeavors to improve their talents and skills.

Gordon B. Hinckley said,

> Marriage, in its truest sense, is a partnership of equals, with neither exercising dominion over the other, but, rather, with each encouraging and assisting the other in whatever responsibilities and aspirations he or she might have.[17]

When we talk about individual growth, we are talking about growth that builds the individual with the purpose of building the family. Almost always, individual growth that serves the family is mental, emotional, and/or spiritual growth.

Individual growth should bring us closer to our spouse and strengthen that relationship.

Both of us grew up with orchards behind our homes. Depending on their growth potential, fruit trees are usually planted between 15 and 30 feet apart so that they have room to mature. As the trees grow, their branches lengthen, and they grow closer to one another. They fill in and make the orchard look complete. As children, we both spent hours in the orchards. The mature trees offered protection from the sun and endless entertainment.

For a Power Couple, individual growth should be patterned after an orchard that starts out with trees planted apart. As time goes by, you are not only growing individually, but also growing together.

Mature parents who have cultivated their lives to grow closer together instead of apart are reminiscent of those thriving orchards we loved. The unified confidence and strength of those parents provides a safe, protected place for their children to explore and grow their own interests and talents.

Some people separate themselves from their spouse (whether intentionally or not) in the name of "individual growth" by pursuing hobbies and activities that increasingly take them away from their family. When you become caught up in any culture that competes with and detracts from your most important relationships, it can become a selfish endeavor and a difficult trap to escape.

One Power Couple we know has really exemplified the principle of growing together. Melinda and Ryan were introduced to the growing sport of pickleball and started playing a few nights a week after putting their kids to bed. They both took naturally to it and Melinda's background as a college tennis player helped her advance quickly in the game, earn a sponsorship, and be able to compete with the top players in the world.

However, despite a love of the game and a fiercely competitive nature, Melinda realized that playing at that level wasn't really aligned with her purpose in life and she made the difficult decision to step back. Melinda said:

> When it became too competitive and time-consuming it became more of a burden than fun. I felt like I always had to practice and play at a high level so playing "for fun" wasn't fun anymore. At times I felt like I had to make a choice between family and pickleball. Family would/should always win, so I stopped pursuing it.[18]

Melinda continues to play pickleball, but primarily for fun. She and Ryan love to play together for date night, or as doubles partners in the local league, where it has also been a great segue into new friendships. She is happy to keep her tournament schedule local and have pickleball serve as a hobby that builds her relationships...and nets an occasional sponsorship.

Mutual Growth

In our observations, the strongest couples learn to support and enjoy each other's interests and hobbies, turning them into something that not only builds the individual, but also the relationship.

Exploring new hobbies together and finding a new common ground can add another dimension to your relationship. Whether it is pickleball, hiking, thrifting, or competitive dog grooming(!), if you do it together it's likely to invite more joy into your marriage.

Kevin Rathunde, a family and consumer studies professor at the University of Utah is quoted in a Chicago Tribune Article as saying,

People dismiss 'hobbies' as an old-fashioned word, but these are the things that make us human and creative (…) When family members learn a hobby together, they share what they love with people they love.[19]

Dr. Arthur Aron, a social psychology professor at State University of New York, has conducted both observational and controlled studies demonstrating that new and exciting experiences together (skiing, hiking, dancing, and challenge exercises are some examples given) show a significant increase in marital satisfaction compared with mundane or typical date night activities.[20]

It's important to note that we certainly do not advocate renouncing all personal hobbies or friends, but rather that you stay mindful of the tipping point when activities or friendships move from offering positive contributions to your ultimate goals and when they become distractions.

Understanding your purpose in life and weighing all things against it will help you keep perspective and know what should take priority in your life.

All growth depends upon activity.

NEW HABIT FORMATION
Write down the habit you would like to incorporate, including when you will do it. Whenever possible, pair the desired habit with an existing habit. For situational habits designate an if...then clause.

EXAMPLES

- Study scriptures together and discuss for 20 minutes every evening before bed.

- Find and try a new hike together each Saturday morning.

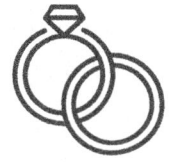

HABIT #5

WORK TOGETHER TOWARDS GOALS

Make and review couple and family goals and help each other be accountable.

WORK TOGETHER TOWARDS GOALS

Most couples have several undefined and unspoken goals that they are already working towards. Power couples work towards focused, clearly defined and clearly outlined short-term and long-term goals.

Accountability Partners

We had some great friends, Jordan and Shayna, in the early years of our marriage that were very driven and goal oriented. After losing touch for several years, Scott's residency program took us to Texas, where Jordan and Shayna were also living, and we had an opportunity to catch up.

It was so great to walk into their bedroom and see that they were still going strong on their goal setting. The evidence was right there on the wall, in the form of a massive whiteboard right across from their bed. Their goals and the steps to reaching them were laid out clearly, with reminders and inspirational quotes to spur them on. We were so impressed by this obvious commitment to working together to achieve greatness.

It's said that one of the highest indicators of success in goal setting is to tell somebody about your goal so that you are accountable. When you and your spouse act as accountability partners and remind each other daily that you have common goals, positive results come faster.

Long-Term Goals

Frequently discussing your long-term goals keeps them in the forefront of your mind. Then when difficulties arise that might make a less motivated couple lose sight of their goals, you will be able to focus, allowing you to sidestep the roadblocks and continue your journey.

We all have situations where we have varying opinions on how to proceed or when one spouse does or says something differently than we would have. However, when you know that you have the same ultimate goal, it's easier to let go of those small differences in execution and hang on to what matters most.

Short-Term Goals

Short-term goals cement your relationship day-by-day, leading you to the successful completion of your long-term goals that you can enjoy together.

A team that wins together is able to build trust and gain momentum. Short-term goals are those quick wins that cement your team and give you the desire to keep working together. The quick wins help defend against discouragement, especially when it seems like long-term goals are far away.

A colleague and clinical social worker, Iuri Melo said, "Be less concerned about the velocity with which you are traveling, and more focused on the vector of your travels."

Break your big goals down into smaller goals. Monthly, yearly, whatever it may be. Maybe your long-term goal is to sell your home in five years and spend a year traveling before you settle back down into a smaller retirement home. Break that down into small supporting goals and work together on projects to increase your home's value. Redo your bathroom, update your flooring, and plant some perennials. Spend time together researching where you want to travel. Good planning allows you to work on your short-term goals together in a less stressful way.

AMY'S PARENTS, Terry and Marguerite, have been a strong example and reminder of how working together towards goals builds a relationship.

We'd like to end this section with their example. When asked to share how short-term goals have helped them achieve their long-term goals and how this process has united their marriage, Terry said:

Like many couples, we came from rather disparate backgrounds. Our individual life experiences in youth and childhood did not have a lot in common. Though our level of education was similar, the subject matter differed. Our work and vocational experiences varied considerably as well. And, of course, there were the understandable differences of perspective and preference inherent to gender. These and many other challenges had to be dealt with if we were to become united and compatible in our marriage.

For most couples, agreeing upon long-term goals is typically not a large problem. Most couples at least begin the marriage wanting to "live happily ever after." But it is important to define what that means for each partner.

We were in agreement that, for us, "happily ever after" meant quickly beginning our family; which would include quite a few children. We wanted to make our family a higher priority than our occupations. Our religious faith and devotion to God would also be a top priority. We did not seek to become particularly wealthy, but it was important to us to live comfortably and to provide our children with an excellent education and a safe, secure home in a wholesome neighborhood.

We desired for all of our children to become self-reliant by gaining a university education, participating in educational and humanitarian service away from home before marriage and then marrying well so they could begin families of their own. We also desired for them to become independent from us in their spiritual commitments and practices.

We really did not consider many long-term goals beyond these at that time. Now we recognize that we should have looked beyond our years of parenting dependent children to the years ahead when we would live only as a couple again.

Now, let us look at the role that short-term goals play in enabling the long-term goals to be more easily agreed upon. Let us also consider the challenges of reaching unity in making the necessary short-term goals.

We began our marriage with both of us working full time in our separate careers. Neither of us earned enough individually to support a family in the manner we desired. However, our long-term goals unified us and strengthened our resolve in such a way that we could make sacrifices in the short term. This mutually agreed-upon strategy greatly diminished the pain and contention often resulting from sacrifice.

In order to save and prepare for our future family, we agreed to forego having a nice apartment or home with comfortable amenities. Instead, we would be contented with our one-bedroom basement apartment until we had two children living in that single room with us.

We also decided that we would prepare all our own meals rather than going out to eat. We made some of our own baby food instead of buying only the convenient, commercially prepared products.

Please understand that it is not our intent to advocate our short-term strategies as the plan others should adopt, even for similar long-term goals. We only wish to illustrate that our long-term goals gave us the strength and unity to employ what we viewed as necessary short-term goals without harming our happiness.

Our long-term goals also helped us make a decision about where our income would need to be generated as our family grew. I, the husband, truly desired for our children to have a full-time mother at home. This was becoming less and less common in society and less and less attainable.

Marguerite loved her career as an elementary school teacher. I knew that I would have to at least double my earnings in sales and business to enable our first child to have her full-time mother. It was my short-term goal to make that happen during the first year of our marriage. Then, we would at least have the desired option when the day of parenthood arrived for us.

I achieved my short-term goal! When my wife held that precious little daughter in her arms at the end of our first year of marriage, it was not hard for her to put her career on hold for the foreseeable future in order for her to become a full-time mother. In fact, her experience in elementary education made her very qualified for this career change. Her career change also made many more of our long-term goals more attainable.

I also made an important career decision at that time which proved to be of great importance in attaining some of our long-term priorities; the decision to be home with my family each evening and weekend.

We had another ambitious medium-term goal and that was to build our own home for our family. I had worked my way through college in the home construction industry. Though my chosen career and education was in business, we really wanted to design and build our own home. This goal really helped to unify us through those years of personal sacrifice while our children were yet young. We thought it better to sacrifice while they were too young to compare their lives and possessions with other children.

We discussed ideas together, looked at homes and neighborhoods, drew up plans, and soon settled on purchasing a building lot in an area that fit our long-term goals. We began making payments so our lot could be paid for in full before we began construction. It took great discipline, but we did it, and saved an additional amount so as to qualify for our construction loan. There was no "easy money" to be borrowed at that time, when interest rates were around 14%.

These years of extreme sacrifice, when money was very tight and recreation was rare, when we were working long hours and welcomed a new member of the family every two years were, perhaps, the happiest years of our lives. The reason for this was that we had our goals clearly in mind, we were working in unity with all our might to accomplish them and we were making steady and measurable progress.

It would be less than honest to say that we never disagreed nor had some serious arguments. We can both be quite stubborn in the defense of our opinions. Weariness and fatigue can certainly take a toll on a marriage like this when there are so many competing needs and priorities demanding both time and money. Personal weaknesses originating in the experiences of youth and childhood can, unfortunately, place impediments in our way, making unhindered progress towards our goals quite impossible from time to time. Yet, when there is an eternal commitment to the marriage covenant and an underlying commitment to mutual long-term goals, power can be found to press on through the temporary and very real times of despair until we emerge again out of the darkness and into the light.

We realized recently that we had not given much thought to long-term goals beyond raising our children to independence. We decided that it was time to look to the future once again and make some new goals.

Fortunately, we had not ignored the need to save and invest in our post retirement future. Our principal investments were these: our health, our children, our home, our business and our retirement accounts. These investments enabled us to have some precious options which all too few people enjoy at this stage of life.

We both feel that we owe a great debt to God for the blessings which we have received at his hand by the grace of our Lord, Jesus Christ. We feel that our present circumstances are a direct result of our attempts to apply the gospel of Jesus Christ in our lives. Now we have decided together to embark on a new era of personal sacrifice and service to others in order to demonstrate our gratitude to God.

Last year, we decided that we could and should sell our business, our home, and most of our belongings so we could become missionaries and take the message of the restored gospel of Jesus Christ to people and places where it is needed. We felt it to be safe to entrust our family into God's hands and we accepted a call to serve the people of the small town of Sibu, on the island of Borneo, in East Malaysia.

This is an exciting time of life for us. We now spend virtually all our time together as a couple in the service of God and our fellow beings. It is almost like the first years of our marriage in that we are learning and experiencing things never before encountered.

We have rediscovered the reasons why we chose each other as partners in the first place. We have extracted ourselves from the plateaus of complacency and security which so easily entrap people of our age, so that we may begin to climb new mountains and discover latent abilities within ourselves which we were previously not utilizing.

The synergy of unity in our partnership has replaced the—sometimes selfish—tendency towards finding fulfillment on diverging tracks. We have found that we can do almost anything together. We are learning to let go of anxiety and to accept the challenges that come to us as we meet them.

We do not know all that shall happen to us in the sunset of our lives, but we trust that the same strategy which got us to this point will see us through to the end.

Make and review couple and family goals and help each other be accountable.

NEW HABIT FORMATION

Write down the habit you would like to incorporate, including when you will do it. Whenever possible, pair the desired habit with an existing habit. For situational habits designate an if...then clause.

EXAMPLES

• Make a goal or vision board and update it monthly

• Set aside time each Sunday evening to review our week together. Discuss progress on short term goals and assess current habits to see if they support our goals. Add new habits as necessary.

FINAL
THOUGHTS

Are you
willing to do
what it takes
to create a
life that you
love?

IN CONCLUSION

STEP OUTSIDE OF YOUR DAY, your week, and your month for a minute and look with a bigger perspective. Who are you right now and who can you become? Physical, mental, and spiritual issues can hold us back. What's holding you back from becoming an even better version of your already amazing self?

We believe that we are all children of God. Because we believe in an all-knowing and all-powerful God as our greatest example of how to live life, we need to elevate our expectations of what is possible for us. The pattern of parenthood is to raise children to become like their parents and we believe that our Heavenly Father has more in mind for us than we can begin to comprehend. When we believe that we have the innate capacity to follow in His footsteps and become like Him, everything changes.

We begin to tap into that potential by transforming our mindset, by learning from those who have gone before us and those who shine around us, and by optimizing our brains and our bodies through cutting-edge science that God has inspired.

There is incredible power in partnering with someone who can lovingly encourage you to elevate your personal expectations.

This is the origin story of every true Power Couple and the gateway to continuous growth and endless potential.

REFERENCES

INTRODUCTION

1 Anand, P., Kunnumakara, A. B., Sundaram, C., Harikumar, K. B., Tharakan, S. T., Lai, O. S., ... & Aggarwal, B. B. (2008). Cancer is a preventable disease that requires major lifestyle changes. Pharmaceutical research, 25(9), 2097-2116.w

2 Garrett, J. Personal Communication, April 18, 2019

3 Covey, S. R. (1989). The 7 Habits of Highly Effective People

4 Hardy, B. (2019, February 22). 35 Hard Truths You Should Know Before Becoming "Successful". Retrieved from https://medium.com/thrive-global/35-hard-truths-you-should-know-before-becoming-successful-4f146ac40899

....

Section 1: NUTRITION

1 Merrill, R. M., Aldana, S. G., Pope, J. E., Anderson, D. R., Coberley, C. R., Grossmeier, J. J., & Whitmer, R. W. (2013). Self-Rated Job Performance and Absenteeism According to Employee Engagement, Health Behaviors, and Physical Health. Journal of Occupational and Environmental Medicine, 55(1), 10-18. doi:10.1097/jom.0b013e31827b73af

2 Durstine, J.L., Gordon, B., Zhengzhen W., Xijuan L., (2013). Chronic disease and the link to physical activity. Journal of Sport and Health Science, 2 (1), 3-11. doi:10.1016/j.jshs.2012.07.009.

3 Allison, R. L. (2017). Back to Basics: The Effect of Healthy Diet and Exercise on Chronic Disease Management. Retrieved from https://www.ncbi.nlm.nih.gov/pubmed/28817856

4 Fardet, A., & Boirie, Y. (2014). Associations between food and beverage groups and major diet-related chronic diseases: An exhaustive review of pooled/meta-analyses and systematic reviews. Nutrition Reviews,72(12), 741-762. doi:10.1111/nure.12153

5   Kimokoti, R. W., & Millen, B. E. (2016, November). Nutrition for the Prevention of Chronic Diseases. Retrieved from https://www.ncbi.nlm.nih.gov/pubmed/27745589#

6   JAMA and Archives Journals. (2009, August 12). Healthy Lifestyle Habits May Be Associated With Reduced Risk Of Chronic Disease. ScienceDaily. Retrieved April 12, 2019 from www.sciencedaily.com/releases/2009/08/090810161906.htm

7   Brown, K., DeCoffe, D., Molcan, E., & Gibson, D. L. (n.d.). Diet-induced dysbiosis of the intestinal microbiota and the effects on immunity and disease. Retrieved from https://www.ncbi.nlm.nih.gov/pmc/articles/PMC3448089/

8   https://www.melissaclark.net/books

9   Volkow, N. D., Wang, G. J., Fowler, J. S., Tomasi, D., & Baler, R. (2012). Food and drug reward: Overlapping circuits in human obesity and addiction. Retrieved from https://www.ncbi.nlm.nih.gov/pubmed/22016109

10   Moss, M. (2013, February 20). The Extraordinary Science of Addictive Junk Food. Retrieved from https://www.nytimes.com/2013/02/24/magazine/the-extraordinary-science-of-junk-food.html

11   Swithers, S. E. (2013, September). Artificial sweeteners produce the counterintuitive effect of inducing metabolic derangements. Retrieved from https://www.ncbi.nlm.nih.gov/pubmed/23850261

12   Permission to share stories has been recieved and names have been changed.

13   Stopping any medication abruptly is not recommended. Please consult your physician before starting or stopping any medication.

14   Worthington, V. (1998, January). Effect of agricultural methods on nutritional quality: A comparison of organic with conventional crops. Retrieved from https://www.ncbi.nlm.nih.gov/pubmed/9439021

15   Dean, A., & Armstrong, J. (2009, May 9). Genetically Modified Foods. Retrieved from http://www.aaemonline.org/gmo.php

16   Bohn, T., Cuhra, M., Traavik, T., Sanden, M., Fagan, J., & Primicerio, J. (2013, December 18). Compositional differences in soybeans on the market: Glyphosate accumulates in Roundup Ready GM soybeans. Retrieved from https://www.sciencedirect.com/science/article/pii/S0308814613019201

17   Ponder, J. (2019, February 20). School of Public Health study links unhealthy diet to mental illness in California adults. Retrieved from https://news.llu.edu/research/school-of-public-health-study-links-unhealthy-diet-mental-illness-california-adults

18   Banta, J. E., Segovia-Siapco, G., Crocker, C. B., Montoya, D., & Alhusseini, N.
      (n.d.). Mental health status and dietary intake among California adults: A popula-
      tion-based survey. Retrieved from https://www.tandfonline.com/doi/full/10.1080/09
      637486.2019.1570085

19   Simões-Wüst, A. P., Moltó-Puigmartí, C., Jansen, E. H., Van Dongen, M. C.,
      Dagnelie, P. C., & Thijs, C. (2017, August). Organic food consumption during
      pregnancy and its association with health-related characteristics: The KOALA Birth
      Cohort Study. Retrieved from https://www.ncbi.nlm.nih.gov/pubmed/28625206

20   Alfvén, T., Braun-Fahrländer, C., Brunekreef, B., Von Mutius, E., Riedler, J.,
      Scheynius, A., . . . PARSIFAL study group. (2006, April). Allergic diseases and
      atopic sensitization in children related to farming and anthroposophic lifestyle--the
      PARSIFAL study. Retrieved from https://www.ncbi.nlm.nih.gov/pubmed/16512802

21   Rist, L., Mueller, A., Barthel, C., Snijders, B., Jansen, M., Simões-Wüst, A. P., .
      . . Thijs, C. (2007, April). Influence of organic diet on the amount of conjugated
      linoleic acids in breast milk of lactating women in the Netherlands. Retrieved from
      https://www.ncbi.nlm.nih.gov/pubmed/17349086

22   Stenius, F., Swartz, J., Lilja, G., Borres, M., Bottai, M., Pershagen, G., . . .
      Alm, J. (2011, June 09). Lifestyle factors and sensitization in children – the
      ALADDIN birth cohort. Retrieved from https://onlinelibrary.wiley.com/doi/
      abs/10.1111/j.1398-9995.2011.02662.x

23   Fagerstedt, S., Hesla, H. M., Ekhager, E., Rosenlund, H., Mie, A., Benson, L., .
      . . Alm, J. (2016). Anthroposophic lifestyle is associated with a lower incidence
      of food allergen sensitization in early childhood. Journal of Allergy and Clinical
      Immunology, 137(4). doi:10.1016/j.jaci.2015.11.009

24   Alm, J. S., Swartz, J., Lilja, G., Scheynius, A., & Pershagen, G. (1999). Atopy in
      children of families with an anthroposophic lifestyle. The Lancet, 353(9163), 1485-
      1488. doi:10.1016/s0140-6736(98)09344-1

25   Flöistrup, H., Swartz, J., Bergström, A., Alm, J. S., Scheynius, A., Van Hage, M., . . .
      Parsifal Study Group. (2006, January). Allergic disease and sensitization in Steiner
      school children. Retrieved from https://www.ncbi.nlm.nih.gov/pubmed/16387585

26   Kummeling, I., Thijs, C., Huber, M., Van de Vijver, L. P., Snijders, B. E., Penders, J.,
      . . . Dagnelie, P. C. (2008, March). Consumption of organic foods and risk of atopic
      disease during the first 2 years of life in the Netherlands. Retrieved from https://
      www.ncbi.nlm.nih.gov/pubmed/17761012

27   Kesse-Guyot, E., Baudry, J., Assmann, K. E., Galan, P., Hercberg, S., & Lairon,
      D. (2017, January). Prospective association between consumption frequency of
      organic food and body weight change, risk of overweight or obesity: Results
      from the NutriNet-Santé Study. Retrieved from https://www.ncbi.nlm.nih.gov/
      pubmed/28166859

28   Kesse-Guyot, E., Péneau, S., Méjean, C., Szabo de Edelenyi, F., Galan, P., Hercberg, S., & Lairon, D. (2013, October 18). Profiles of organic food consumers in a large sample of French adults: Results from the Nutrinet-Santé cohort study. Retrieved from https://www.ncbi.nlm.nih.gov/pubmed/24204721

29   Baudry, J., Méjean, C., Péneau, S., Galan, P., Hercberg, S., Lairon, D., & Kesse-Guyot, E. (2015, December 28). Health and dietary traits of organic food consumers: Results from the NutriNet-Santé study. Retrieved from https://www.ncbi.nlm.nih.gov/pubmed/26429066

30   Bae, S., & Hong, Y. (2015, February). Exposure to bisphenol A from drinking canned beverages increases blood pressure: Randomized crossover trial. Retrieved from https://www.ncbi.nlm.nih.gov/pubmed/25489056#

31   Rudel, R. A., Gray, J. M., Engel, C. L., Rawsthorne, T. W., Dodson, R. E., Ackerman, J. M., . . . Brody, J. G. (2011, July 01). Food packaging and bisphenol A and bis(2-ethyhexyl) phthalate exposure: Findings from a dietary intervention. Retrieved from https://www.ncbi.nlm.nih.gov/pmc/articles/PMC3223004/

32   Kaume, L., Howard, L. R., & Devareddy, L. (2011, November 14). The Blackberry Fruit: A Review on Its Composition and Chemistry, Metabolism and Bioavailability, and Health Benefits. Retrieved from https://pubs.acs.org/doi/abs/10.1021/jf203318p

33   Wunderlich, S. M., Feldman, C., Kane, S., & Hazhin, T. (2008, February). Nutritional quality of organic, conventional, and seasonally grown broccoli using vitamin C as a marker. Retrieved from https://www.ncbi.nlm.nih.gov/pubmed/1785 2499?ordinalpos=1&itool=EntrezSystem2.PEntrez.Pubmed.Pubmed_ResultsPanel. Pubmed_DefaultReportPanel.Pubmed_RVDocSum

34   Watters, C. (2013, August). The Nutrition Benefits of Eating Locally. Retrieved from https://www.ctahr.hawaii.edu/sustainag/news/articles/V16-Watters-BenefitsLocalFood.pdf

35   The biggest spending category for food eaten at home is "miscellaneous," which requires some further explanation, as it doesn't actually suggest much home "cooking." This category appears to be comprised mostly of premade meals and snacks (think Hot Pockets and Lean Cuisines, as well as Doritos and almonds), though it also includes: "condiments and seasonings, such as olives, pickles, relishes, sauces and gravies, baking needs and other specified condiments; and other canned and packaged prepared foods, such as salads, desserts, baby foods, and vitamin supplements."

     Morrell, A. (2017, February 17). A close look at Americans' food budget shows an obvious place to save money. Retrieved from https://www.businessinsider.com/americans-spending-food-bls-2017-2

CONSUMER EXPENDITURES MIDYEAR UPDATE--JULY 2016 THROUGH JUNE 2017 AVERAGE. (2018, April 26). Retrieved from https://www.bls.gov/news.release/cesmy.nr0.htm

https://www.bls.gov/cex/csxgloss.htm#chars

36 Doctrine and Covenants 38. (n.d.). Retrieved from https://www.lds.org/scriptures/dc-testament/dc/38.30?lang=eng

37 Laska, M. N., Larson, N. I., Neumark-Sztainer, D., & Story, M. (2012, July). Does involvement in food preparation track from adolescence to young adulthood and is it associated with better dietary quality? Findings from a 10-year longitudinal study. Retrieved from https://www.ncbi.nlm.nih.gov/pubmed/22124458

38 Appelhans, B. M., Waring, M. E., Schneider, K. L., & Pagoto, S. L. (2014, May). Food preparation supplies predict children's family meal and home-prepared dinner consumption in low-income households. Retrieved from https://www.ncbi.nlm.nih.gov/pubmed/24462491

39 Rettner, R. (2010, August 05). Brain's Link Between Sounds, Smells and Memory Revealed. Retrieved from https://www.livescience.com/8426-brain-link-sounds-smells-memory-revealed.html

40 Giray, C., & Ferguson, G. M. (2018, September 01). Say yes to "Sunday Dinner" and no to "Nyam and Scram": Family mealtimes, nutrition, and emotional health among adolescents and mothers in Jamaica. Retrieved from https://www.ncbi.nlm.nih.gov/pubmed/29803778

41 Larson, N., Fulkerson, J., Story, M., & Neumark-Sztainer, D. (2013, May). Shared meals among young adults are associated with better diet quality and predicted by family meal patterns during adolescence. Retrieved from https://www.ncbi.nlm.nih.gov/pubmed/22857517

42 Larson, N. I., Neumark-Sztainer, D., Hannan, P. J., & Story, M. (2007, September). Family meals during adolescence are associated with higher diet quality and healthful meal patterns during young adulthood. Retrieved from https://www.ncbi.nlm.nih.gov/pubmed/17761227

43 Laska, M. N., Hearst, M. O., Lust, K., Lytle, L. A., & Story, M. (2015, August). How we eat what we eat: Identifying meal routines and practices most strongly associated with healthy and unhealthy dietary factors among young adults. Retrieved from https://www.ncbi.nlm.nih.gov/pubmed/25439511

44 Berge, J. M., Truesdale, K. P., Sherwood, N. E., Mitchell, N., Heerman, W. J., Barkin, S., . . . French, S. A. (2017, December). Beyond the dinner table: Who's having breakfast, lunch and dinner family meals and which meals are associated with better diet quality and BMI in pre-school children? Retrieved from https://www.ncbi.nlm.nih.gov/pubmed/28903804

45   Suggs, L. S., Della Bella, S., Rangelov, N., & Marques-Vidal, P. (2018, February 01).
     Is it better at home with my family? The effects of people and place on children's
     eating behavior. Retrieved from https://www.ncbi.nlm.nih.gov/pubmed/29122583

46   National Turkey Neck Soup Day is March 30th, if you didn't already know.

47   Vik, F. N., Bjørnarå, H. B., Overby, N. C., Lien, N., Androutsos, O., Maes, L., . . .
     Bere, E. (2013, May 15). Associations between eating meals, watching TV while
     eating meals and weight status among children, ages 10-12 years in eight European
     countries: The ENERGY cross-sectional study. Retrieved from https://www.ncbi.
     nlm.nih.gov/pubmed/23675988

48   Avery, A., Anderson, C., & McCullough, F. (2017, October). Associations between
     children's diet quality and watching television during meal or snack consumption: A
     systematic review. Retrieved from https://www.ncbi.nlm.nih.gov/pubmed/28211230

49   Varady, K. A. (2016, October). Meal frequency and timing: Impact on metabolic
     disease risk. Retrieved from https://www.ncbi.nlm.nih.gov/pubmed/27455514

50   Kogevinas, M., Espinosa, A., Castelló, A., Gómez-Acebo, I., Guevara, M., Martin,
     V., . . . Romaguera, D. (2018, November 15). Effect of mistimed eating patterns on
     breast and prostate cancer risk (MCC-Spain Study). Retrieved from https://www.
     ncbi.nlm.nih.gov/pubmed/30016830

51   Falco, M., Wyant T., et al. Lifetime Risk of Developing or Dying From Cancer.
     (n.d.). Retrieved from https://www.cancer.org/cancer/cancer-basics/lifetime-proba-
     bility-of-developing-or-dying-from-cancer.html

52   Yoshino, W., B., Okunade, Imai, Shin-ichiro, Mittendorfer, . . . Samuel. (2014,
     September 01). Diurnal Variation in Insulin Sensitivity of Glucose Metabolism
     Is Associated With Diurnal Variations in Whole-Body and Cellular Fatty Acid
     Metabolism in Metabolically Normal Women. Retrieved from https://academic.oup.
     com/jcem/article/99/9/E1666/2537471

53   Wehrens, S. M., Christou, S., Isherwood, C., Middleton, B., Gibbs, M. A., Archer,
     S. N., . . . Johnston, J. D. (2017, June 19). Meal Timing Regulates the Human
     Circadian System. Retrieved from https://www.ncbi.nlm.nih.gov/pubmed/28578930

54   St-Onge, M., Ard, J., Baskin, M. L., Chiuve, S. E., Johnson, H. M., Kris-Etherton, P.,
     . . . American Heart Association Obesity Committee of the Council on Lifestyle and
     Cardiometabolic Health; Council on Cardiovascular Disease in the Young; Council
     on Clinical Cardiology; and Stroke Council. (2017, February 28). Meal Timing
     and Frequency: Implications for Cardiovascular Disease Prevention: A Scientific
     Statement From the American Heart Association. Retrieved from https://www.ncbi.
     nlm.nih.gov/pubmed/28137935

55   Patterson, R. E., & Sears, D. D. (2017, July 17). Metabolic Effects of Intermittent
     Fasting. Retrieved from https://www.annualreviews.org/doi/full/10.1146/

annurev-nutr-071816-064634?url_ver=Z39.88-2003&rfr_id=ori:rid:crossref.
org&rfr_dat=cr_pub=pubmed

56   Sutton, E., Beyl, R., Early, K., Cefalu, W., Ravussin, E., & Peterson, C. (2018, May
      10). Early Time-Restricted Feeding Improves Insulin Sensitivity, Blood Pressure,
      and Oxidative Stress Even without Weight Loss in Men with Prediabetes. Retrieved
      from https://www.sciencedirect.com/science/article/pii/S1550413118302535

57   Tello, M. (2018, June 26). Intermittent fasting: Surprising up-
      date. Retrieved from https://www.health.harvard.edu/blog/
      intermittent-fasting-surprising-update-2018062914156

58   Aubrey, A. (2017, October 02). How Messing With Our Body
      Clocks Can Raise Alarms With Health. Retrieved from https://
      www.npr.org/sections/health-shots/2017/10/02/555054483/
      how-messing-with-our-body-clocks-can-raise-alarms-with-health

59   Nas, A., Mirza, N., Hägele, F., Kahlhöfer, J., Keller, J., Rising, R., ... & Bosy-
      Westphal, A. (2017). Impact of breakfast skipping compared with dinner
      skipping on regulation of energy balance and metabolic risk. The American
      journal of clinical nutrition, 105(6), 1351-1361. https://academic.oup.com/ajcn/
      article/105/6/1351/4668664

60   Horne, B., May, H., Anderson, J., Kfoury, A., Bailey, B., McClure, B., . . .
      Muhlestein, J. (2008, October 01). ClinicalKey. Retrieved from https://www.clini-
      calkey.com/#!/content/playContent/1-s2.0-S0002914908009016?returnurl=https://
      linkinghub.elsevier.com/retrieve/pii/S0002914908009016?showall=true&referrer=

61   Teachings of Ezra Taft Benson pp. 476-7. Retrieved from http://media.ldscdn.org/
      pdf/scripture-and-lesson-support/teachings-of-presidents-of-the-church-ezra-taft-
      benson/2015-01-00-teachings-of-presidents-of-the-church-ezra-taft-benson-eng.pdf

62   Enstrom, J. E. (2006, June 29). Cancer and total mortality among ac-
      tive mormons. Retrieved from https://onlinelibrary.wiley.com/doi/
      abs/10.1002/1097-0142(197810)42:43.0.CO;2-L

63   New Archive Reveals How the Food Industry Mimics Big Tobacco to Suppress
      Science, Shape Public Opinion. (2018, December 05). Retrieved from https://civile-
      ats.com/2018/11/28/new-archive-reveals-how-the-food-industry-mimics-big-tobacc-
      to-suppress-science-shape-public-opinion/?_ke=eyJrbF9lbWFpbCI6ICJhbXlub29yZ
      GFAZ21haWwuY29tIiwgImtsX2NvbXBhbnlfaWQiOiAibXk3NXk2In0=

64   Ensign, September 1988, p. 5. Retrieved from https://www.churchofjesuschrist.org/
      study/ensign/1988/09/in-his-steps?lang=eng

65   van der Plaat, D. A., de Jong, K., de Vries, M., van Diemen, C. C., Nedeljković, I.,
      Amin, N., ... & Boezen, H. M. (2018). Occupational exposure to pesticides is associ-
      ated with differential DNA methylation. Occup Environ Med, 75(6), 427-435.https://
      oem.bmj.com/content/75/6/427

66   Mnif, W., Hassine, A. I. H., Bouaziz, A., Bartegi, A., Thomas, O., & Roig, B. (2011). Effect of endocrine disruptor pesticides: a review. International journal of environmental research and public health, 8(6), 2265-2303. https://www.ncbi.nlm.nih.gov/pmc/articles/PMC3138025/

67   Benson, E. T. (n.d.). Do Not Despair. Retrieved from https://www.lds.org/general-conference/1974/10/do-not-despair?lang=eng

68   Cannon, G. Q. (n.d.). Word of Wisdom-Fish Culture-Dietetics. Retrieved from http://jod.mrm.org/12/221

....

Section 2: SLEEP

1   CDC Newsroom. (2016). Retrieved from https://www.cdc.gov/media/releases/2016/p0215-enough-sleep.html

2   https://www.cnn.com/2018/10/25/success/arianna-huffington-sleep-thrive/index.html

3   Leaf, C. (2016, November 30). Dream Catcher. Retrieved from http://fortune.com/arianna-huffington-thrive-global-company/

4   Hafner, Marco, Stepanek, Martin, Taylor, Jirka, . . . Christian. (2016, November 30). Sleep Deprivation Has Economic, Physical, and Social Consequences. Retrieved from https://www.rand.org/pubs/research_reports/RR1791.html

5   Watson, Buchwald, Jj, Vitiello, Noonan, Gharib, & Nf. (2017, January 25). Transcriptional Signatures of Sleep Duration Discordance in Monozygotic Twins. Retrieved from https://academic.oup.com/sleep/article/40/1/zsw019/2952682

6   Kitamura, S., Katayose, Y., Nakazaki, K., Motomura, Y., Oba, K., Katsunuma, R., . . . Mishima, K. (2016, October 24). Estimating individual optimal sleep duration and potential sleep debt. Retrieved from https://www.ncbi.nlm.nih.gov/pmc/articles/PMC5075948/

7   Watson, N. F., Badr, M. S., Belenky, G., Bliwise, D. L., Buxton, O. M., Buysse, D., . . . Tasali, E. (2015, June 01). Recommended Amount of Sleep for a Healthy Adult: A Joint Consensus Statement of the American Academy of Sleep Medicine and Sleep Research Society. Retrieved from https://www.ncbi.nlm.nih.gov/pmc/articles/PMC4434546/

8   Schmid, S. M., Hallschmid, M., Jauch-Chara, K., & Schultes, B. (2008, June 28). A single night of sleep deprivation increases ghrelin levels and feelings of hunger in normal-weight healthy men. Retrieved from https://onlinelibrary.wiley.com/doi/full/10.1111/j.1365-2869.2008.00662.x

9   Nackerdien, Z. (2018, December 9). Oversleeping May Up Heart Disease, Death Risks - Multinational PURE study presents new analyses of sleep patterns. Retrieved from https://www.medpagetoday.com/sso-token.php?redirecturl=/cardiology/prevention/76798?xid=nl_mpt_DHE_2018-12-12&eun=g1021534d0r&pos=1111111 &utm_term=NL_Daily_DHE_Active

10   Reilly, T. (1990). Human circadian rhythms and exercise. Retrieved from https://www.ncbi.nlm.nih.gov/pubmed/2286092

11   Mirsky, S. (2017, October 02). Nobel Prize Explainer: Circadian Rhythm's Oscillatory Control Mechanism. Retrieved from https://www.scientificamerican.com/podcast/episode/nobel-prize-explainer-circadian-rhythms-oscillatory-control-mechanism/

12   Mirsky, S. (2017, October 02). Nobel Prize Explainer: Circadian Rhythm's Oscillatory Control Mechanism. Retrieved from https://www.scientificamerican.com/podcast/episode/nobel-prize-explainer-circadian-rhythms-oscillatory-control-mechanism/

13   Masters, J. (2017, October 02). US body clock scientists win Nobel prize. Retrieved from https://www.cnn.com/2017/10/02/health/nobel-medicine-prize-circadian-rhythm/index.html

14   Plihal, W., & Born, J. (1999, September 01). Effects of early and late nocturnal sleep on priming and spatial memory | Psychophysiology. Retrieved from https://www.cambridge.org/core/journals/psychophysiology/article/effects-of-early-and-late-nocturnal-sleep-on-priming-and-spatial-memory/1DF290C59947C821E85674843B9 8D157

15   Gais, S., Plihal, W., Wagner, U., & Born, J. (2000, December 01). Early sleep triggers memory for early visual discrimination skills. Retrieved from https://www.nature.com/articles/nn1200_1335

16   Plihal, W., & Born, J. (2008, January 07). Effects of Early and Late Nocturnal Sleep on Declarative and Procedural Memory. Retrieved from https://www.mitpressjournals.org/doi/abs/10.1162/jocn.1997.9.4.534

17   Figueiro, M., Steverson, B., Heerwagen, J., Kampschroer, K., Hunter, C., Gonzalez, K., . . . Rea, M. (2017). The impact of daytime light exposures on sleep and mood in office workers. Sleep Health,3(3), 204-215. doi:10.1016/j.sleh.2017.03.005

18   Doctrine and Covenants 88. (n.d.). Retrieved February 01, 2019, from https://www.lds.org/scriptures/dc-testament/dc/88.118?lang=eng

19   Merz, B. (2016, September 08). Resetting your circadian clock to minimize jet lag. Retrieved from https://www.health.harvard.edu/blog/resetting-your-circadian-clock-to-minimize-jet-lag-2016090810279

20 Wehrens, S. M., Christou, S., Isherwood, C., Middleton, B., Gibbs, M. A., Archer, S. N., . . . Johnston, J. D. (2017, June 19). Meal Timing Regulates the Human Circadian System. Retrieved from https://www.ncbi.nlm.nih.gov/pubmed/28578930

21 Herxheimer, A., & Petrie, K. J. (2002). Melatonin for the prevention and treatment of jet lag. Retrieved from https://www.ncbi.nlm.nih.gov/pubmed/12076414

22 Bauducco, S., Flink, I., Jansson-Fröjmark, M., & Linton, S. (2016, August 11). Sleep duration and patterns in adolescents: Correlates and the role of daily stressors. Retrieved from http://oru.diva-portal.org/smash/record.jsf?pid=diva2:952069&dsw id=-1967

23 Lunsford-Avery, J. R., Engelhard, M. M., Navar, A. M., & Kollins, S. H. (2018, September 21). Validation of the Sleep Regularity Index in Older Adults and Associations with Cardiometabolic Risk. Retrieved from https://www.nature.com/articles/s41598-018-32402-5#Abs1

24 Breus, M. (2014, June 12). Junk sleep: When sleep and technology don't mix. Retrieved from https://www.cnn.com/2014/06/12/health/junk-sleep-live-longer/index.html

25 Harvard Health Publishing. (2012, May). Blue light has a dark side. Retrieved from https://www.health.harvard.edu/staying-healthy/blue-light-has-a-dark-side

26 Burkhart, K., & Phelps, J. R. (2009, December). Amber lenses to block blue light and improve sleep: A randomized trial. Retrieved from https://www.ncbi.nlm.nih.gov/pubmed/20030543

27 University of Haifa. (2017, August 22). Blue light emitted by screens damages our sleep, study suggests. ScienceDaily. Retrieved April 16, 2019 from www.sciencedaily.com/releases/2017/08/170822103434.htm

28 Hysing, M., Pallesen, S., Stormark, K. M., Jakobsen, R., Lundervold, A. J., & Sivertsen, B. (2015, January 01). Sleep and use of electronic devices in adolescence: Results from a large population-based study. Retrieved from https://bmjopen.bmj.com/content/5/1/e006748

29 Christensen, M. A., Bettencourt, L., Kaye, L., Moturu, S. T., Nguyen, K. T., Olgin, J. E., . . . Marcus, G. M. (2016, November 09). Direct Measurements of Smartphone Screen-Time: Relationships with Demographics and Sleep. Retrieved from https://www.ncbi.nlm.nih.gov/pubmed/27829040

30 Stevens, R. G. (2016, June 17). American Medical Association warns of health and safety problems from 'white' LED streetlights. Retrieved from http://theconversation.com/american-medical-association-warns-of-health-and-safety-problems-from-white-led-streetlights-61191

31 Chamorro, E., Bonnin-Arias, C., Pérez-Carrasco, M. J., Muñoz de Luna, J., Vázquez, D., & Sánchez-Ramos, C. (2013, March). Effects of light-emitting diode radiations on human retinal pigment epithelial cells in vitro. Retrieved from https://www.ncbi.nlm.nih.gov/pubmed/22989198

32 Gooley, J. J., Chamberlain, K., Smith, K. A., Khalsa, S. B., Rajaratnam, S. M., Van Reen, E., . . . Lockley, S. W. (2011, March). Exposure to room light before bedtime suppresses melatonin onset and shortens melatonin duration in humans. Retrieved from https://www.ncbi.nlm.nih.gov/pmc/articles/PMC3047226/

33 Park, Y. M. M., White, A. J., Jackson, C. L., Weinberg, C. R., & Sandler, D. P. (2019). Association of Exposure to Artificial Light at Night While Sleeping With Risk of Obesity in Women. JAMA internal medicine.

34 Obradovich, N., Migliorini, R., Mednick, S. C., & Fowler, J. H. (2017, May 26). Nighttime temperature and human sleep loss in a changing climate. Retrieved from https://www.ncbi.nlm.nih.gov/pmc/articles/PMC5446217/

35 Okamoto-Mizuno, K., & Mizuno, K. (2012, May 31). Effects of thermal environment on sleep and circadian rhythm. Retrieved from https://www.ncbi.nlm.nih.gov/pmc/articles/PMC3427038/

36 P. Strøm-Tejsen, P., Zukowska, D., Wargocki, P., & Wyon, D. P. (2015, October 09). The effects of bedroom air quality on sleep and next-day performance. Retrieved from https://onlinelibrary.wiley.com/doi/full/10.1111/ina.12254#ina12254-bib-0010

37 Messineo, L., Taranto-Montemurro, L., Sands, S. A., Oliveira Marques, M. D., Azabarzin, A., & Wellman, D. A. (2017, December 21). Broadband Sound Administration Improves Sleep Onset Latency in Healthy Subjects in a Model of Transient Insomnia. Retrieved from https://www.ncbi.nlm.nih.gov/pmc/articles/PMC5742584/

38 Claudio, L. (2011, October 1). Planting healthier indoor air. Retrieved from https://www.ncbi.nlm.nih.gov/pmc/articles/PMC3230460/

39 https://www.jscimedcentral.com/SleepMedicine/sleepmedicine-2-1022.pdf

40 Kim, W., & Hur, M. H. (2016, December). Inhalation Effects of Aroma Essential Oil on Quality of Sleep for Shift Nurses after Night Work. Retrieved from https://www.ncbi.nlm.nih.gov/pubmed/28077825

41 Lillehei, A. S., & Halcon, L. L. (2014, June). A systematic review of the effect of inhaled essential oils on sleep. Retrieved from https://www.ncbi.nlm.nih.gov/pubmed/24720812

42 Lillehei, A. S., Halcón, L. L., Savik, K., & Reis, R. (2015, July 01). Effect of Inhaled Lavender and Sleep Hygiene on Self-Reported Sleep Issues: A Randomized Controlled Trial. Retrieved from https://www.ncbi.nlm.nih.gov/pubmed/26133206

43 Ayik, C., & Özden, D. (2018, February). The effects of preoperative aromatherapy massage on anxiety and sleep quality of colorectal surgery patients: A randomized controlled study. Retrieved from https://www.ncbi.nlm.nih.gov/pubmed/29458940

44 Lee, Y., Wu, Y., Tsang, H. W., Leung, A. Y., & Cheung, W. M. (2011, February). A systematic review on the anxiolytic effects of aromatherapy in people with anxiety symptoms. Retrieved from https://www.ncbi.nlm.nih.gov/pubmed/21309711

45 Dyer, J., Cleary, L., McNeill, S., Ragsdale-Lowe, M., & Osland, C. (2016, February). The use of aromasticks to help with sleep problems: A patient experience survey. Retrieved from https://www.ncbi.nlm.nih.gov/pubmed/26850806

46 Harmat, L., Takács, J., & Bódizs, R. (2008, May). Music improves sleep quality in students. Retrieved from https://www.ncbi.nlm.nih.gov/pubmed/18426457

47 Abeln, V., Kleinert, J., Strüder, H. K., & Schneider, S. (2013, July 18). Brainwave entrainment for better sleep and post-sleep state of young elite soccer players - a pilot study. Retrieved from https://www.ncbi.nlm.nih.gov/pubmed/23862643

48 Padmanabhan, R., Hildreth, A. J., & Laws, D. (2005, July 07). A prospective, ran-domised, controlled study examining binaural beat audio and pre-operative anxiety in patients undergoing general anaesthesia for day case surgery*. Retrieved from https://onlinelibrary.wiley.com/doi/full/10.1111/j.1365-2044.2005.04287.x

49 Huang, T., & Charyton, C. (1970, January 01). A comprehensive review of the psy-chological effects of brainwave entrainment. Retrieved from https://www.ncbi.nlm.nih.gov/books/NBK75019/

50 Smith, L. (2017, November 14). Binaural beats therapy: Benefits and how they work. Retrieved from https://www.medicalnewstoday.com/articles/320019.php

51 Reynolds, G. (2015, May 20). Lack of Exercise Can Disrupt the Body's Rhythms. Retrieved from https://well.blogs.nytimes.com/2015/05/20/lack-of-exercise-can-disrupt-the-bodys-rhythms/

52 Reilly, T. (1990). Human circadian rhythms and exercise. Retrieved from https://www.ncbi.nlm.nih.gov/pubmed/2286092

53 Harrington, M. E. (2012, December 01). Exercise strengthens circadian clocks. Retrieved from https://www.ncbi.nlm.nih.gov/pmc/articles/PMC3530104/

54 Wright Jr., K. P., McHill, A. W., Birks, B. R., Griffin, B. R., Rusterholz, T., & Chinoy, E. D. (2013). Entrainment of the Human Circadian Clock to the Natural Light-Dark Cycle. Current Biology, 23(16), 1554-1558. doi:10.1016/j.cub.2013.06.039

55 Bulletproof Staff. (2017, December 12). Does Grounding Really Work? Retrieved from https://blog.bulletproof.com/does-grounding-work/

56 Cryan, J. F., & O'Mahony, S. M. (2011, February 08). The microbiome-gut-brain axis: From bowel to behavior. Retrieved from https://onlinelibrary.wiley.com/doi/full/10.1111/j.1365-2982.2010.01664.x

57 Ramakrishna, B. S. (2013, December). Role of the gut microbiota in human nutrition and metabolism. Retrieved from https://www.ncbi.nlm.nih.gov/pubmed/24251697

58 Benedict, C., Vogel, H., Jonas, W., Woting, A., Blaut, M., Schurmann, A., & Cedernaes, J. (2016, October 24). Gut microbiota and glucometabolic altera-tions in response to recurrent partial sleep deprivation in normal-weight young individuals. Retrieved from https://www.sciencedirect.com/science/article/pii/S2212877816301934

59 Anderson, J. R., Carroll, I., Azcarate-Peril, M. A., Rochette, A. D., Heinberg, L. J., Peat, C., . . . Gunstad, J. (2017, October). A preliminary examination of gut micro-biota, sleep, and cognitive flexibility in healthy older adults. Retrieved from https://www.ncbi.nlm.nih.gov/pubmed/29031742

60 Takada, M., Nishida, K., Kataoka-Kato, A., Gondo, Y., Ishikawa, H., Suda, K., . . . Rokutan, K. (2016, July). Probiotic Lactobacillus casei strain Shirota relieves stress-associated symptoms by modulating the gut-brain interaction in human and animal models. Retrieved from https://www.ncbi.nlm.nih.gov/pubmed/26896291

61 News & Announcements. (2008, May 22). Retrieved from https://sleep.med.harvard.edu/news/229/Harvard study finds fasting resets circadian clock

62 Drake, C., Roehrs, T., Shambroom, J., & Roth, T. (2013). Caffeine Effects on Sleep Taken 0, 3, or 6 Hours before Going to Bed. Journal of Clinical Sleep Medicine. doi:10.5664/jcsm.3170

63 Alcoholism: Clinical & Experimental Research. (2013, January 22). Reviewing alcohol's effects on normal sleep. ScienceDaily. Retrieved April 16, 2019 from www.sciencedaily.com/releases/2013/01/130122162236.htm

64 Roehrs, T., & Roth, T. (n.d.). ALCOHOL ALERT. Retrieved from https://pubs.niaaa.nih.gov/publications/arh25-2/101-109.htm

65 Chan, J. K., Trinder, J., Colrain, I. M., & Nicholas, C. L. (2015, January 16). The Acute Effects of Alcohol on Sleep Electroencephalogram Power Spectra in Late Adolescence. Retrieved from https://onlinelibrary.wiley.com/doi/abs/10.1111/acer.12621

66 Afshar, M. K., Moghadam, Z. B., Taghizadeh, Z., Bekhradi, R., Montazeri, A., & Mokhtari, P. (2015). Lavender fragrance essential oil and the quality of sleep in post-partum women. Iranian Red Crescent Medical Journal, 17(4). Retrieved from https://www.ncbi.nlm.nih.gov/pmc/articles/PMC4443384/

67 Goel, N., Kim, H., & Lao, R. P. (2005). An olfactory stimulus modifies nighttime

sleep in young men and women. Chronobiology International, 22(5), 889-904. Retrieved from https://www.tandfonline.com/doi/abs/10.1080/07420520500263276

68 University of Washington Health Sciences / UW Medicine. (2017, November 22). Chronic Sleep Deprivation Suppresses Immune System. Retrieved from https://www.infectioncontroltoday.com/immune-system/chronic-sleep-deprivation-suppresses-immune-system

69 Patke, A., Murphy, P. J., Onat, O. E., Krieger, A. C., Özçelik, T., Campbell, S. S., & Young, M. W. (2017). Mutation of the human circadian clock gene CRY1 in familial delayed sleep phase disorder. Cell, 169(2), 203-215. https://www.cell.com/cell/fulltext/S0092-8674(17)30346-X

70 Haridy, R. (2017, April 10). Can't get to sleep? The reason may be in your genes. Retrieved from https://newatlas.com/gene-explains-night-owl-sleep/48902/

71 Sorensen, E. (2017, April 05). 'Sleep gene' offers clues about why we need our zzzs | WSU Insider | Washington State University. Retrieved from https://news.wsu.edu/2017/04/05/sleep-gene-why-we-need-our-zzzs/

....

Section 3: STRESS

1 Bridgewater, L. C., Zhang, C., Wu, Y., Hu, W., Zhang, Q., Wang, J., . . . Zhao, L. (2017). Gender-based differences in host behavior and gut microbiota composition in response to high fat diet and stress in a mouse model. Scientific Reports, 7(1). doi:10.1038/s41598-017-11069-4

2 Kresser, Chris. (2019, February 12). The little-known key to a healthy gut. https://chriskresser.com/

3 Echouffo-Tcheugui, J. B., Conner, S. C., Himali, J. J., Maillard, P., Decarli, C. S., Beiser, A. S., . . . Seshadri, S. (2018). Circulating cortisol and cognitive and structural brain measures. Neurology, 91(21). doi:10.1212/wnl.0000000000006549

4 Dort, I. (2017). *Thinking & Acting With A Compassionate Heart: Principles And Ideas That Unlock The Human Potential* [Kindle DX version]. Retrieved from Amazon.com

5 Moreno-Smith, M., Lutgendorf, S. K., & Sood, A. K. (2010). Impact of stress on cancer metastasis. Future oncology, 6(12), 1863-1881. https://www.ncbi.nlm.nih.gov/pmc/articles/PMC3037818/

6 Mantovani, A., Allavena, P., Sica, A., & Balkwill, F. (2008). Cancer-related inflammation. Nature, 454(7203), 436. https://www.nature.com/articles/nature07205

7 Powell, N. D., Tarr, A. J., & Sheridan, J. F. (2013). Psychosocial stress and inflammation in cancer. Brain, behavior, and immunity, 30, S41-S47. https://www.ncbi.nlm.nih.gov/pubmed/22790082

8 Payne, J. K. (2014, September). State of the science: stress, inflammation, and cancer. In Oncology nursing forum (Vol. 41, No. 5). https://www.ncbi.nlm.nih.gov/pubmed/25158658

9 Tofield, A. (2014, April). Stress and myocardial infarction. Retrieved from https://www.ncbi.nlm.nih.gov/pubmed/24818229 https://www.ncbi.nlm.nih.gov/pubmed/24818229

10 Alcántara, C., Muntner, P., Edmondson, D., Safford, M. M., Redmond, N., Colantonio, L. D., & Davidson, K. W. (2015). Perfect storm: concurrent stress and depressive symptoms increase risk of myocardial infarction or death. Circulation: Cardiovascular Quality and Outcomes, 8(2), 146-154. https://www.ncbi.nlm.nih.gov/pubmed/25759443

11 Consoli, S. M. (2015). Occupational stress and myocardial infarction. Presse medicale (Paris, France: 1983), 44(7-8), 745-751. https://www.ncbi.nlm.nih.gov/pubmed/26150284

12 Stuller, K. A., Jarrett, B., & DeVries, A. C. (2012). Stress and social isolation increase vulnerability to stroke. Experimental neurology, 233(1), 33-39. https://www.ncbi.nlm.nih.gov/pubmed/21281636

13 Kotlęga, D., Gołąb-Janowska, M., Masztalewicz, M., Ciećwież, S., & Nowacki, P. (2016). The emotional stress and risk of ischemic stroke. Neurologia i neurochirurgia polska, 50(4), 265-270. https://www.ncbi.nlm.nih.gov/pubmed/27375141

14 Wagenmaker, E. R., Breen, K. M., Oakley, A. E., Pierce, B. N., Tilbrook, A. J., Turner, A. I., & Karsch, F. J. (2009). Cortisol interferes with the estradiol-induced surge of luteinizing hormone in the ewe. Biology of reproduction, 80(3), 458-463.https://www.ncbi.nlm.nih.gov/pmc/articles/PMC2805396/

15 Viau, V. (2002). Functional cross-talk between the hypothalamic-pituitary-gonadal and-adrenal axes. Journal of neuroendocrinology, 14(6), 506-513. https://onlinelibrary.wiley.com/doi/abs/10.1046/j.1365-2826.2002.00798.x

16 Divine Discontent, Michelle D. Craig, First Counselor in the Young Women's General Presidency. The Church of Jesus Christ of Latter-Day Saints. October 2018. Retrieved from https://www.churchofjesuschrist.org/study/general-conference/2018/10/divine-discontent?lang=eng

17   Oaks, D. H. (n.d.). Good, Better, Best. Speech. Retrieved April 16, 2019, from https://www.lds.org/general-conference/2007/10/good-better-best?lang=eng

18   Cunningham, L. (2012, October 03). Exhaustion is not a status symbol. Retrieved from https://www.washingtonpost.com/national/exhaustion-is-not-a-status-symbol/2012/10/02/19d27aa8-0cba-11e2-bb5e-492c0d30bff6_story.html?noredirect=on&utm_term=.2175624fe997

19   McKeown, G. (2014). Essentialism: The disciplined pursuit of less. New York: Crown Business. https://gregmckeown.com/book/

20   Keith, N. R. (2013). Tidier homes, fitter bodies? Retrieved from http://newsinfo.iu.edu/web/page/normal/14627.html

21   Saxbe DE1, Repetti R. No place like home: home tours correlate with daily patterns of mood and cortisol. Pers Soc Psychol Bull. 2010 Jan;36(1):71-81. doi: 10.1177/0146167209352864. Epub 2009 Nov 23.

22   National Sleep Foundation. (2011). Bedroom Poll: Summary of Findings. Retrieved January 15, 2019, from https://www.sleepfoundation.org/sites/default/files/inline-files/NSF_Bedroom_Poll_Report.pdf

23   The Healing Power of Forgiveness, James E. Faust, Second Counselor in the First Presidency. The Church of Jesus Christ of Latter-Day Saints. April 2007. https://www.lds.org/study/general-conference/2007/04/the-healing-power-of-forgiveness?lang=eng

24   Forget Me Not, Dieter F. Uchtdorf, Second Counselor in the First Presidency. The Church of Jesus Christ of Latter-Day Saints. October 2011. Retrieved from https://www.lds.org/general-conference/2011/10/forget-me-not?lang=eng

25   Rajanala, S., Maymone, M. B., & Vashi, N. A. (2018). Selfies—living in the era of filtered photographs. JAMA facial plastic surgery, 20(6), 443-444. https://jamanetwork.com/journals/jamafacialplasticsurgery/article-abstract/2688763

26   Su'a, J. (2015, October 23). The Power of Pausing. Retrieved from https://www.linkedin.com/pulse/power-pausing-justin-su-a/

27   Su'a, J. (2015, June 05). TEDx Talks - Learn how to use time-outs in life | Justin Su'a | TEDxYouth@IMGAcademy. Retrieved from https://www.youtube.com/watch?v=LYzuqhBU0Ic

     Transcription edited for clarity by Justin Su'a in personal interview on 28 Feb. 2019

28   Connie, E., Froerer, A., Von Cziffra-Bergs, J., & Kim, J. (2018, August 21). Solution-Focused Brief Therapy with Clients Managing Trauma. https://www.amazon.com/Solution-Focused-Therapy-Clients-Managing-Trauma/dp/019067878X

29 Kyu HH, Bachman VF, Alexander LT, et al. Physical activity and risk of breast cancer, colon cancer, diabetes, ischemic heart disease, and ischemic stroke events: Systematic reviews and dose-response meta-analysis for the Global Burden of Disease Study 2013. [Published online ahead of print August 9, 2016]. BMJ. doi:10.1136/bmj.i3857.

30 Esch T, Stefano GB. Endogenous reward mechanisms and their importance in stress reduction, exercise and the brain. Arch Med Sci. 2010; 6 (3): 447–55. https://www.ncbi.nlm.nih.gov/pmc/articles/PMC3282525/

31 Greenwood BN, Fleshner M. Exercise, stress resistance, and central serotonergic systems. Exerc Sport Sci Rev. 2011; 39 (3): 140–9. https://www.ncbi.nlm.nih.gov/pmc/articles/PMC4303035/

32 Hamilton MT, Healy GN, Dunstan DW, Zderic TW, Owen N. Too Little Exercise and Too Much Sitting: Inactivity Physiology and the Need for New Recommendations on Sedentary Behavior. Current cardiovascular risk reports. 2008;2(4):292-298. doi:10.1007/s12170-008-0054-8. https://link.springer.com/article/10.1007/s12170-008-0054-8 https://link.springer.com/article/10.1007/s12170-008-0054-8

33 Shilpa Dogra and Liza Stathokostas, "Sedentary Behavior and Physical Activity Are Independent Predictors of Successful Aging in Middle-Aged and Older Adults," Journal of Aging Research, vol. 2012, Article ID 190654, 8 pages, 2012. doi:10.1155/2012/190654 https://www.hindawi.com/journals/jar/2012/190654/abs/ https://www.hindawi.com/journals/jar/2012/190654/abs/

34 Ellingson LD, Shields MR, Stegner AJ, Cook DB. Physical activity, sustained sedentary behavior, and pain modulation in women with fibromyalgia. J Pain. 2012 Feb;13(2):195-206. https://www.sciencedirect.com/science/article/pii/S1526590011008716

35 de Rezende, L. F. M., Lopes, M. R., Rey-López, J. P., Matsudo, V. K. R., & do Carmo Luiz, O. (2014). Sedentary behavior and health outcomes: an overview of systematic reviews. PloS one, 9(8), e105620 https://journals.plos.org/plosone/article?id=10.1371/journal.pone.0105620

36 Chong CSM, Tsunaka M, Tsang HWH, Chan EP, Cheung WM. Effects of yoga on stress management in healthy adults: a systematic review. Altern Ther Health Med. 2011; 17 (1): 32–8. https://search.proquest.com/openview/25de198b92bec3b56b7f6e9f60630ea5/1?pq-origsite=gscholar&cbl=32528

37 Melville GW, Chang D, Colagiuri B, Marshall PW, Cheema BC. Fifteen minutes of chair-based yoga postures or guided meditation performed in the office can elicit a relaxation response. Evid Based Complement Alternat Med [Internet]. 2012 https://www.hindawi.com/journals/ecam/2012/501986/abs/

38 Li AW, Goldsmith CW. The effects of yoga on anxiety and stress. Altern Med Rev. 2012; 17 (1): 21–35. https://web.b.ebscohost.com/abstract?direct=true&profile=ehost &scope=site&authtype=crawler&jrnl=10895159&AN=75210880&h=jqQyw2tyU%2 bv84VmWe8WSv9jK8jyPz%2bEg1oyf3GCc2f7e5BpFDRrkVSJ02NR80M6WrBNI O5KRDRWCV3smZDSPUg%3d%3d&crl=c&resultNs=AdminWebAuth&resultLoca l=ErrCrlNotAuth&crlhashurl=login.aspx%3fdirect%3dtrue%26profile%3dehost%26s cope%3dsite%26authtype%3dcrawler%26jrnl%3d10895159%26AN%3d75210880

39 Wang WC, Zhang AL, Rasmussen B, et al.. The effect of Tai Chi on psychological well-being: a systematic review of randomized controlled trials. J Acupunct Meridian Stud. 2009; 2 (3): 171–81. https://www.sciencedirect.com/science/article/pii/ S2005290109600522

40 Young, Simon N. "How to increase serotonin in the human brain without drugs." Journal of psychiatry & neuroscience: JPN 32, no. 6 (2007): 394. https:// www.ncbi.nlm.nih.gov/pmc/articles/PMC2077351/ https://www.ncbi.nlm.nih.gov/ pmc/articles/PMC2077351/

41 Klepeis, N. E., Nelson, W. C., Ott, W. R., Robinson, J. P., Tsang, A. M., Switzer, P., ... & Engelmann, W. H. (2001). The National Human Activity Pattern Survey (NHAPS): a resource for assessing exposure to environmental pollutants. Journal of Exposure Science and Environmental Epidemiology, 11(3), 231. https://www.nature.com/ articles/7500165

42 University of Exeter. (2019, June 13). Two hours a week is key dose of nature for health and wellbeing. ScienceDaily. Retrieved July 3, 2019 from www.sciencedaily. com/releases/2019/06/190613095227.htm https://www.nature.com/articles/7500165

43 Kondo, M. C., Jacoby, S. F., & South, E. C. (2018). Does spending time outdoors reduce stress? A review of real-time stress response to outdoor environments. Health & place, 51, 136-150. https://www.ncbi.nlm.nih.gov/pubmed/29604546 https://www. sciencedirect.com/science/article/abs/pii/S1353829217307633

44 van der Rhee, H., Coebergh, J. W., & de Vries, E. (2009). Sunlight, vitamin D and the prevention of cancer: a systematic review of epidemiological studies. European journal of cancer prevention, 18(6), 458-475. https://www.ncbi.nlm.nih.gov/ pubmed/19730382

45 University of Southampton. (2014, January 17). Here comes the sun to lower your blood pressure. ScienceDaily. Retrieved April 22, 2019 from www.sciencedaily.com/ releases/2014/01/140117090139.htm

46 Young, K. A., Engelman, C. D., Langefeld, C. D., Hairston, K. G., Haffner, S. M., Bryer-Ash, M., & Norris, J. M. (2009). Association of plasma vitamin D levels with adiposity in Hispanic and African Americans. The Journal of Clinical Endocrinology & Metabolism, 94(9), 3306-3313. https://www.ncbi.nlm.nih.gov/pubmed/19549738

47 Walch, J. M., Rabin, B. S., Day, R., Williams, J. N., Choi, K., & Kang, J. D. (2005). The effect of sunlight on postoperative analgesic medication use: a prospective study of patients undergoing spinal surgery. Psychosomatic medicine, 67(1), 156-163.

48 Harvard Health Publishing. (n.d.). 6 things you should know about vitamin D. Retrieved from https://www.health.harvard.edu/ staying-healthy/6-things-you-should-know-about-vitamin-d

49 Wharton, B., & Bishop, N. (2003). Rickets. The Lancet, 362(9393), 1389-1400 https://www.ncbi.nlm.nih.gov/pubmed/14585642?dopt=Abstract

50 Woelk, H., & Schläfke, S. (2010). A multi-center, double-blind, randomised study of the Lavender oil preparation Silexan in comparison to Lorazepam for general- ized anxiety disorder. Phytomedicine, 17(2), 94-99. https://www.sciencedirect.com/ science/article/pii/S094471130900261X

51 Bradley, B. F., Brown, S. L., Chu, S., & Lea, R. W. (2009). Effects of orally admin- istered lavender essential oil on responses to anxiety-provoking film clips. Human Psychopharmacology: Clinical and Experimental, 24(4), 319-330.https://onlinelibrary. wiley.com/doi/abs/10.1002/hup.1016 https://onlinelibrary.wiley.com/doi/abs/10.1002/ hup.1016

52 Chen, M. C., Fang, S. H., & Fang, L. (2015). The effects of aromatherapy in relieving symptoms related to job stress among nurses. International journal of nursing prac- tice, 21(1), 87-93. https://onlinelibrary.wiley.com/doi/abs/10.1111/ijn.12229

53 Seyyed-Rasooli, A., Salehi, F., Mohammadpoorasl, A., Goljaryan, S., Seyyedi, Z., & Thomson, B. (2016). Comparing the effects of aromatherapy massage and inhalation aromatherapy on anxiety and pain in burn patients: A single-blind randomized clini- cal trial. Burns, 42(8), 1774-1780. https://www.sciencedirect.com/science/article/abs/ pii/S0305417916301863

54 Chen, P. J., Chou, C. C., Yang, L., Tsai, Y. L., Chang, Y. C., & Liaw, J. J. (2017). Effects of aromatherapy massage on pregnant women's stress and immune function: A longitudinal, prospective, randomized controlled trial. The Journal of Alternative and Complementary Medicine, 23(10), 778-786. https://www.liebertpub.com/doi/ abs/10.1089/acm.2016.0426

55 Cruz, A. B., TaeHo, K., & SangBum, P. (2010). Effects of lavender (lavandula angustifolia Mill.) and peppermint (Mentha cordifolia Opiz.) odors on anxiety and sport skill performance. The Asian International Journal of Life Sciences, 20(2), 323-329. https://www.researchgate.net/profile/Angelita_Cruz/publica- tion/291782897_Effects_of_lavender_Lavandula_angustifolia_Mill_and_pepper- mint_Mentha_cordifolia_Opiz_aromas_on_subjective_vitality_speed_and_agility/ links/5815811b08aeb720f684ba99/Effects-of-lavender-Lavandula-angustifolia-Mill- and-peppermint-Mentha-cordifolia-Opiz-aromas-on-subjective-vitality-speed-and- agility.pdf

56 Liu, S. H., Lin, T. H., & Chang, K. M. (2013). The physical effects of aromatherapy in alleviating work-related stress on elementary school teachers in Taiwan. Evidence-Based Complementary and Alternative Medicine, 2013. https://www.hindawi.com/journals/ecam/2013/853809/abs/

57 Hwang, J. H. (2006). The effects of the inhalation method using essential oils on blood pressure and stress responses of clients with essential hypertension. Journal of Korean Academy of Nursing, 36(7), 1123-1134. https://synapse.koreamed.org/search.php?where=aview&id=10.4040/jkan.2006.36.7.1123&code=1006JKAN&vmode=FULL

58 Watanabe, E., Kuchta, K., Kimura, M., Rauwald, H. W., Kamei, T., & Imanishi, J. (2015). Effects of bergamot (Citrus bergamia (Risso) Wright & Arn.) essential oil aromatherapy on mood states, parasympathetic nervous system activity, and salivary cortisol levels in 41 healthy females. Complementary Medicine Research, 22(1), 43-49. https://www.karger.com/Article/Abstract/380989

59 Chang, S. Y. (2008). Effects of aroma hand massage on pain, state anxiety and depression in hospice patients with terminal cancer. Journal of Korean Academy of Nursing, 38(4), 493-502. https://synapse.koreamed.org/DOIx.php?id=10.4040/jkan.2008.38.4.493

60 Seo, E. Y., Song, J. A., Hur, M. H., Lee, M. K., & Lee, M. S. (2017). Effects of aroma mouthwash on stress level, xerostomia, and halitosis in healthy nurses: A non-randomized controlled clinical trial. European Journal of Integrative Medicine, 10, 82-89. https://www.sciencedirect.com/science/article/abs/pii/S187638201730032X

61 Lee, M. K., Lim, S., Song, J. A., Kim, M. E., & Hur, M. H. (2017). The effects of aromatherapy essential oil inhalation on stress, sleep quality and immunity in healthy adults: Randomized controlled trial. European Journal of Integrative Medicine, 12, 79-86. https://www.sciencedirect.com/science/article/abs/pii/S1876382017300951

62 Wilkinson, S., Aldridge, J., Salmon, I., Cain, E., & Wilson, B. (1999). An evaluation of aromatherapy massage in palliative care. Palliative medicine, 13(5), 409-417. https://journals.sagepub.com/doi/abs/10.1191/026921699678148345

63 Cho, M. Y., Min, E. S., Hur, M. H., & Lee, M. S. (2013). Effects of aromatherapy on the anxiety, vital signs, and sleep quality of percutaneous coronary intervention patients in intensive care units. Evidence-Based Complementary and Alternative Medicine, 2013. https://www.hindawi.com/journals/ecam/2013/381381/abs/

64 Goes, T. C., Antunes, F. D., Alves, P. B., & Teixeira-Silva, F. (2012). Effect of sweet orange aroma on experimental anxiety in humans. The Journal of Alternative and Complementary Medicine, 18(8), 798-804. https://www.liebertpub.com/doi/abs/10.1089/acm.2011.0551

....

Section 4: PURPOSE + COMMITMENT

1   Boyle, P. A., Buchman, A. S., Barnes, L. L., & Bennett, D. A. (2010). Effect of a
     purpose in life on risk of incident Alzheimer disease and mild cognitive impairment
     in community-dwelling older persons. Archives of general psychiatry, 67(3), 304-310.
     https://www.ncbi.nlm.nih.gov/pubmed/20194831/

2   Kim, E. S., Sun, J. K., Park, N., & Peterson, C. (2013). Purpose in life and reduced
     incidence of stroke in older adults:'The Health and Retirement Study'. Journal
     of psychosomatic research, 74(5), 427-432. https://www.ncbi.nlm.nih.gov/
     pubmed/23597331/

3   Kim, E. S., Sun, J. K., Park, N., Kubzansky, L. D., & Peterson, C. (2013). Purpose in
     life and reduced risk of myocardial infarction among older US adults with coronary
     heart disease: a two-year follow-up. Journal of Behavioral Medicine, 36(2), 124-133.
     https://link.springer.com/article/10.1007/s10865-012-9406-4

4   Alimujiang, A., Wiensch, A., Boss, J., Fleischer, N. L., Mondul, A. M., McLean, K.,
     ... & Pearce, C. L. (2019). Association Between Life Purpose and Mortality Among
     US Adults Older Than 50 Years. JAMA network open, 2(5), e194270-e194270.

5   Kim, E. S., Strecher, V. J., & Ryff, C. D. (2014). Purpose in life and use of preventive
     health care services. Proceedings of the National Academy of Sciences, 111(46),
     16331-16336. https://www.pnas.org/content/111/46/16331#ref-23

6   Kaplin, A., & Anzaldi, L. (2015, May). New movement in neuroscience: A purpose-
     driven life. In Cerebrum: the Dana forum on brain science (Vol. 2015). Dana
     Foundation. https://www.ncbi.nlm.nih.gov/pmc/articles/PMC4564234/

7   Greed, Selfishness, and Overindulgence, Joe J. Christensen, of the
     First Quorum of the Seventy. The Church of Jesus Christ of Latter-Day
     Saints. April 1999. https://www.lds.org/study/general-conference/1999/04/
     greed-selfishness-and-overindulgence?lang=eng

8   Alma 43:45. The Book of Mormon. The Church of Jesus Christ of Latter-Day Saints.
     Retrieved from https://www.lds.org/study/scriptures/bofm/alma/43?l=eng&lang=eng

9   Hardy, B. (2019, February 22). 35 Hard Truths You Should Know Before Becoming
     "Successful". Retrieved from https://medium.com/thrive-global/35-hard-truths-you-
     should-know-before-becoming-successful-4f146ac40899

10   Our Sacred Duty to Honor Women, Russell M. Nelson, Quorum of the
     Twelve Apostles. The Church of Jesus Christ of Latter-Day Saints. April

1999. Retrieved from https://www.lds.org/general-conference/1999/04/
our-sacred-duty-to-honor-women?lang=eng

11 Van Tongeren, D. R., Green, J. D., Davis, D. E., Hook, J. N., & Hulsey, T. L. (2016).
Prosociality enhances meaning in life. The Journal of Positive Psychology, 11(3),
225-236. https://www.tandfonline.com/doi/abs/10.1080/17439760.2015.1048814?jou
rnalCode=rpos20

12 If Ye Had Known Me, David A. Bednar, Quorum of the Twelve Apostles. The Church
of Jesus Christ of Latter-Day Saints. Retrieved from October 2016. https://www.lds.
org/general-conference/2016/10/if-ye-had-known-me?lang=eng

13 McCraty, R., Atkinson, M., Tiller, W. A., Rein, G., & Watkins, A. D. (1995). The effects of emotions on short-term power spectrum analysis of heart rate variability. The
American journal of cardiology, 76(14), 1089-1093. https://www.ncbi.nlm.nih.gov/
pubmed/7484873

14 https://www.intelligentchange.com/

15 McCullough, M. E., & Emmons, R. A. (2003). Counting blessings versus burdens:
An experimental investigation of gratitude and subjective well-being in daily
life. Journal of Personality and Social Psychology, 84(2), 377-389. https://www.ncbi.
nlm.nih.gov/pubmed/12585811

16 Redwine, L., Henry, B. L., Pung, M. A., Wilson, K., Chinh, K., Knight, B., ... & Mills,
P. J. (2016). A pilot randomized study of a gratitude journaling intervention on HRV
and inflammatory biomarkers in Stage B heart failure patients. Psychosomatic medicine, 78(6), 667. https://www.ncbi.nlm.nih.gov/pubmed/27187845

17 Digdon, N., & Koble, A. (2011). Effects of constructive worry, imagery distrac-
tion, and gratitude interventions on sleep quality: A pilot trial. Applied Psychology:
Health and Well-Being, 3(2), 193-206. https://onlinelibrary.wiley.com/doi/
abs/10.1111/j.1758-0854.2011.01049.x

18 Connie, E., Froerer, A., Von Cziffra-Bergs, J., & Kim, J. (2018, August 21). Solution-
Focused Brief Therapy with Clients Managing Trauma. https://www.amazon.com/
Solution-Focused-Therapy-Clients-Managing-Trauma/dp/019067878X

19 Crum, A. J., & Langer, E. J. (2007). Mind-set matters: Exercise and the placebo
effect. Psychological Science, 18(2), 165-171. https://www.ncbi.nlm.nih.gov/
pubmed/17425538?_ke=eyJrbF9lbWFpbCI6ICJhbXlub29yZGFAZ21haWwuY29tIi
wgImtsX2NvbXBhbmlfaWQiOiAibXk3NXk2In0%3D

20 Cascio, C. N., O'donnell, M. B., Tinney, F. J., Lieberman, M. D., Taylor, S. E.,
Strecher, V. J., & Falk, E. B. (2015). Self-affirmation activates brain systems associated with self-related processing and reward and is reinforced by future orienta-
tion. Social cognitive and affective neuroscience, 11(4), 621-629. https://www.ncbi.
nlm.nih.gov/pmc/articles/PMC4814782/

21 Adams, AJ. (2009, Dec 03). Seeing Is Believing. Retrieved from
    https://www.psychologytoday.com/us/blog/flourish/200912/
    seeing-is-believing-the-power-visualization

22 Nelson, Russell M., "The Creation," *The Ensign* (2000, May 1). Retrieved from
    https://www.churchofjesuschrist.org/study/ensign/2000/05/the-creation?lang=eng

....

Section 5: RELATIONSHIP

1   Harvard Health Publishing. (2017, June). Can relationships boost longevity
    and well-being? Retrieved from https://www.health.harvard.edu/mental-health/
    can-relationships-boost-longevity-and-well-being

2   Yang, Y. C., Boen, C., Gerken, K., Li, T., Schorpp, K., & Harris, K. M. (2016). Social
    relationships and physiological determinants of longevity across the human life
    span. Proceedings of the National Academy of Sciences, 113(3), 578-583. http://www.
    pnas.org/content/early/2016/01/02/1511085112.

3   Algoe, S. B., Gable, S. L., & Maisel, N. C. (2010). It's the little things: Everyday
    gratitude as a booster shot for romantic relationships. Personal relationships, 17(2),
    217-233. https://onlinelibrary.wiley.com/doi/abs/10.1111/j.1475-6811.2010.01273.x?
    deniedAccessCustomisedMessage=&userIsAuthenticated=false&

4   Algoe, S. B., Kurtz, L. E., & Hilaire, N. M. (2016). Putting the "you" in "thank you"
    examining other-praising behavior as the active relational ingredient in expressed
    gratitude. Social Psychological and Personality Science, 7(7), 658-666. https://www.
    ncbi.nlm.nih.gov/pmc/articles/PMC4988174/

5   Gable, S. L., Gonzaga, G. C., & Strachman, A. (2006). Will you be there for me
    when things go right? Supportive responses to positive event disclosures. Journal
    of personality and social psychology, 91(5), 904. https://www.ncbi.nlm.nih.gov/
    pubmed/17059309

6   Li, X., Cao, H., Zhou, N., Ju, X., Lan, J., Zhu, Q., & Fang, X. (2018). Daily commu-
    nication, conflict resolution, and marital quality in Chinese marriage: A three-wave,
    cross-lagged analysis. Journal of Family Psychology, 32(6), 733. https://www.ncbi.
    nlm.nih.gov/pubmed/29771550#

7   Worthington Jr, E. L., Berry, J. W., Hook, J. N., Davis, D. E., Scherer, M., Griffin, B.
    J., ... & Sharp, C. B. (2015). Forgiveness-reconciliation and communication-conflict-
    resolution interventions versus retested controls in early married couples. Journal of
    Counseling Psychology, 62(1), 14. https://www.ncbi.nlm.nih.gov/pubmed/25264599#

8   The Women In Our Lives, President Gordon B. Hinckley, President. The Church of

Jesus Christ of Latter-Day Saints. October 2004. Retrieved from https://www.lds.org/general-conference/2004/10/the-women-in-our-lives?lang=eng

9   Slow to Anger, President Gordon B. Hinckley, President. The Church of Jesus Christ of Latter-Day Saints. October 2007. Retrieved from https://www.lds.org/general-conference/2007/10/slow-to-anger?lang=eng

10 Weinstein, N., & Ryan, R. M. (2010). When helping helps: autonomous motivation for prosocial behavior and its influence on well-being for the helper and recipient. Journal of personality and social psychology, 98(2), 222. https://www.researchgate.net/publication/41087502_When_Helping_Helps_Autonomous_Motivation_for_Prosocial_Behavior_and_Its_Influence_on_Well-Being_for_the_Helper_and_Recipient

11 Love Your Wife, Jeffrey R. Holland. Quorum of the Twelve Apostles. The Church of Jesus Christ of Latter-Day Saints. October 2004. Retrieved from https://www.lds.org/study/ensign/2014/01/love-your-wife?lang=eng

13 https://www.amazon.com/How-Sweet-Bitter-Soup-Memoir/dp/1631526146/

14 Personal interview 3.16.19

15 Chan, C., & Mogilner, C. (2017). Experiential gifts foster stronger social relationships than material gifts. Journal of Consumer Research, 43(6), 913-931. https://academic.oup.com/jcr/article-abstract/43/6/913/2632328?redirectedFrom=fulltext

16 Sezer, O., Norton, M. I., Gino, F., & Vohs, K. D. (2016). Family rituals improve the holidays. Journal of the Association for Consumer Research, 1(4), 509-526. https://www.journals.uchicago.edu/doi/abs/10.1086/688495

17 Newell, L. D. (n.d.). Traditions A Foundation For Strong families. Retrieved from https://scholarsarchive.byu.edu/cgi/viewcontent.cgi?referer=https://www.google.com/&httpsredir=1&article=1001&context=marriageandfamilies

18 I Believe, Gordon B. Hinckley, First Counselor in the First Presidency. The Church of Jesus Christ of Latter-Day Saints. Aug 1992. Retrieved from https://www.lds.org/study/ensign/1992/08/i-believe?lang=eng

19 Personal interview 2.27.19

20 Mann, L. (2015, May 12). Hobbies and relationships: Bonds strengthen when pursuing pastime together. Retrieved from https://www.chicagotribune.com/lifestyles/sc-fam-0519-family-hobbies-20150512-story.html?int=lat_digitaladshouse_bx-modal_acquisition-subscriber_ngux_display-ad-interstitial_bx-bonus-story_____

21 Parker-Pope, T. (2008, February 12). Reinventing Date Night for Long-Married Couples. Retrieved from https://www.nytimes.com/2008/02/12/health/12well.html

ACKNOWLEDGEMENTS

Our lives, our knowledge, and everything that we could hope to share has been built up by amazing examples all around us. We find great joy in looking back on our journey and recognizing all of the love and learning that has been sent our way by our cohorts in this great test we call life.

We want to acknowledge specifically:

Parents who raised us in the middle of mountain orchards, abundant backyard gardens, and a faith that brings meaning and purpose to everything we do.

Our brothers and sisters, for their support, for all of the things that they continually teach us, and for adventures to remember and look forward to.

Our children, who are excited to explore with us and are patient with our learning curve. They teach us so much about ourselves and inspire us to try to be better every day.

Great minds that have helped us learn important things: Dr. Mark Hyman and The Institute for Functional Medicine. Dr. Chris Kresser, Dr. David Hill, Dr. Mercola, Dr. John Doulliard, Dr. Dale Bredesen, Dr. Kelly Brogan, Dr. Amy Meyers, Norman Doidge, Dr. Josh Axe.

Our editorial team: Lizette Balsdon, for being the first eyes on our book and for her proofreading. Terry Stephens, Laura Snow, and Tammy Chenault, for brilliant editing and counsel.

Pam Baird, for her encouragement and teaching me (Amy) so much about writing.

Chandler Bolt, Lise Cartwright, and their team, for sharing their expertise and giving us direction, confidence, and accountability.

David Harris, Dr. Isaac Jones, Dr. Matt Accurso, and Karen Wojciechowski, for helping us expand our mindsets and break free.

Dr. Brannick Riggs, Ezra Segura, Nate Peck, and the Prime Meridian team, for their partnership and for helping manage our clinic so that we could spend evenings writing.

Above all, we are grateful for our Father in Heaven, our Savior, Jesus Christ, and the golden thread of divine love and direction that has (in retrospect!) stitched our life experiences together so neatly.

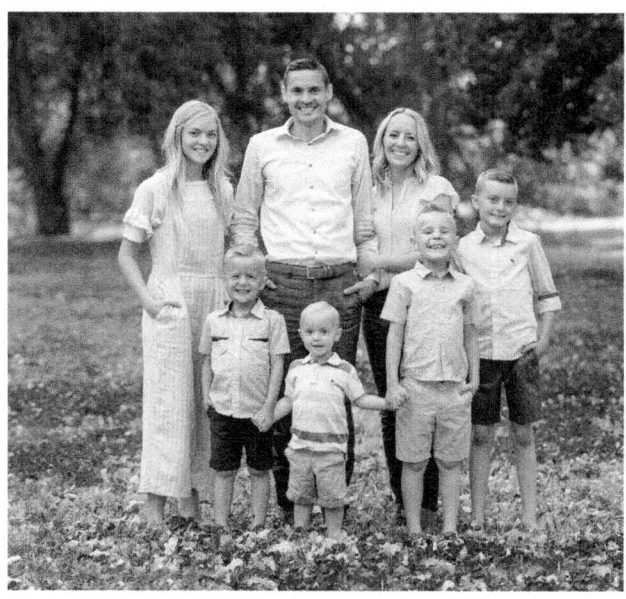

SCOTT NOORDA, DO, studied Neuroscience at Brigham Young University before attending medical school at Midwestern University in Chicago. He is board-certified in Family Medicine. While working for several years with patients with late-stage Alzheimer's and advanced chronic conditions, Dr. Noorda recognized the immense need for preventive care and obtained additional training in Functional Medicine, nutrition, and epigenetics.

AMY NOORDA worked in publishing as a Creative Director and is the magic behind making everything look and sound good. An avid researcher (and superhuman speed reader), she reads and writes extensively on natural health, preventive medicine, and nutrition.

Scott and Amy have five children. They have lived all over the country and enjoy hiking, traveling, and exploring as a family. They love cooking and eating food from different cultures and inviting friends over for impromptu dinners.

Made in the USA
Las Vegas, NV
29 January 2023

66478335R00184